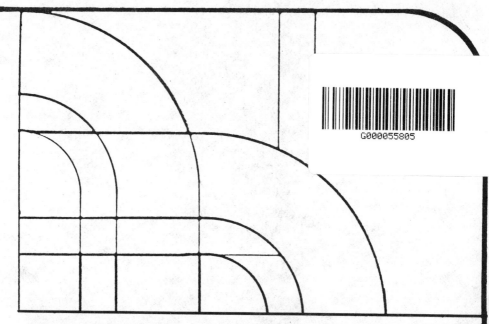

NURSING DIAGNOSIS

JUDITH H. CARLSON, R.N., M.S.N. Associate Professor, Medical-Surgical Nursing
St. Louis University

CAROL A. CRAFT, R.N., M.S. Educational Specialist, South Central
Regional Medical Education Center,
Veterans Hospital, St. Louis, MO
Associate Clinical Professor of Nursing
St. Louis University

ANNE D. McGUIRE, R.N., M.S.N. Former Instructor, Medical-
Surgical Nursing
St. Louis University

W.B. SAUNDERS COMPANY

Philadelphia London Toronto Mexico City Rio de Janeiro Sydney Tokyo

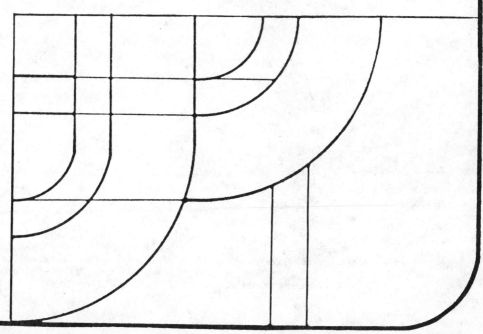

W. B. Saunders Company: West Washington Square
Philadelphia, PA 19105

1 St. Anne's Road
Eastbourne, East Sussex BN21 3UN, England

1 Goldthorne Avenue
Toronto, Ontario M8Z 5T9, Canada

Apartado 26370–Cedro 512
Mexico 4, D.F., Mexico

Rua Coronel Cabrita, 8
Sao Cristovao Caixa Postal 21176
Rio de Janeiro, Brazil

9 Waltham Street
Artarmon, N.S.W. 2064, Australia

Ichibancho, Central Bldg., 22-1 Ichibancho
Chiyoda-Ku, Tokyo 102, Japan

Library of Congress Cataloging in Publication Data

Main entry under title:

Nursing diagnosis.

1. Nursing.   2. Diagnosis.   I. Carlson,
Judith H.   II. Craft, Carol A.   III. McGuire, Anne D.

RT48.N88   616.07'5'024613   81-50272

ISBN 0-7216-2392-1·   AACR2

Nursing Diagnosis   ISBN   0-7216-2392-1

Last digit is the print number: 9   8   7   6   5   4   3

This book is dedicated to:

My Parents — Jeanne and Karl Hockenberger
                      Patricia and Robert Johnson
My Husband — Eddie
My Children — Robert, Mark, Margaret

                                     JUDY

My Parents — Gene and Ida Roach
My Husband — Joe
My Children — Joseph, Jennifer, Michael, Timothy

                                     CAROL

My Parents — Dallas and Eunice Dyer
My Husband — Michael
My Child — Megan

                                  ANNE

CONTRIBUTORS

ANN MARIE BECKER, R.N., M.S.N.
Associate Professor, Saint Louis University School of Nursing, Saint Louis, Missouri

JUDITH H. CARLSON, R.N., M.S.N.
Associate Professor, Medical-Surgical Nursing, Saint Louis University School of Nursing, Saint Louis, Missouri

PATRICIA M. CERONE, R.N., M.S.N.
Former Adjunct Assistant Professor, Saint Louis University School of Nursing, Saint Louis, Missouri

CAROL A. CRAFT, R.N., M.S.
Educational Specialist, South Central Regional Medical Education Center, Veterans Administration, Saint Louis, Missouri; Associate Clinical Professor of Nursing, Saint Louis University School of Nursing, Saint Louis, Missouri

PATRICIA L. DEMUTH, R.N., Ph.D.
Professor of Nursing, Saint Louis University School of Nursing, Saint Louis, Missouri

HELEN R. DiCROCE, R.N., B.S.N., M.S.N.
Associate Professor, Chairman Nursing of Children, Saint Louis University School of Nursing, Saint Louis, Missouri

MARGIE EDEL, R.N., M.S.N.
Adjunct Assistant Professor of Graduate Medical-Surgical Nursing, Saint Louis University School of Nursing, Saint Louis, Missouri

MARY ELLEN GROHAR, R.N., M.S.N., Doctoral Candidate
Assistant Professor of Nursing, Saint Louis University School of Nursing, Saint Louis, Missouri

JOAN HRUBETZ, R.N., Ph.D.
Associate Professor of Nursing, Assistant Dean for Students, Saint Louis University School of Nursing, Saint Louis, Missouri

ANNE D. McGUIRE, R.N., M.S.N.
Former Instructor in Nursing, Saint Louis University School of Nursing, Saint Louis, Missouri

RUTH BECKMANN MURRAY, R.N., M.S.N.
Professor, Psychiatric Nursing and Assistant Dean, Continuing Nursing Education, Saint Louis University School of Nursing, Saint Louis, Missouri

ANNE GRIFFIN PERRY, R.N., M.S.N.
Assistant Professor of Nursing and Coordinator, Respiratory Option, Graduate Medical-Surgical Nursing Major, Saint Louis University School of Nursing, Saint Louis, Missouri

CORDIE GIVEN REESE, R.N., M.S.N.
Associate Professor of Nursing, Saint Louis University School of Nursing; Cardiovascular Clinical Specialist, Saint Louis University Doctors' Office Building, Saint Louis, Missouri

MARION M. RESLER, R.N., M.S.N.
Assistant Professor of Nursing, Saint Louis University School of Nursing, Saint Louis, Missouri

MARILYN E. RICKETTS, R.N., M.S.N.
Assistant Professor, Saint Louis University School of Nursing, Saint Louis, Missouri

MARGUERITE ROBY, R.N., B.S.N., M.S.N.
Professor of Nursing, Saint Louis University School of Nursing, Saint Louis, Missouri

MARILYN B. RUBIN, R.N., Ph.D.
Professor of Nursing, Saint Louis University School of Nursing, Saint Louis, Missouri

DOROTHY E. SASSENRATH, R.N., M.S.
Educational Specialist Long Term Care, South Central Regional Medical Education Center, Veterans Administration, Saint Louis, Missouri; Associate Clinical Professor, Saint Louis University School of Nursing, Saint Louis, Missouri

FLORENCE STELZER, R.N., M.S.N.
Assistant Professor, Saint Louis University School of Nursing, Saint Louis, Missouri

CAROL M. VIAMONTES, R.N., M.S.N.
Former Instructor in Nursing, Saint Louis University School of Nursing, Saint Louis, Missouri; Clinical Nurse, Memorial Sloan-Kettering Cancer Center, New York, New York

FOREWORD

In 1973, I had the pleasure of co-chairing the First National Conference on the Classification of Nursing Diagnosis. In the months of preparation for that session it became obvious that while many nurses intuited the need for and use of nursing diagnoses in practice, little had been put in writing. Communication was occurring by word of mouth among small clusters of nurses working in specific settings or with certain groups of clients.

The forces acting upon nursing in the 1970's made it clear that no group of health care providers could expect increased public support, increased professional respect, or increased monetary reward unless that group was known to have a direct impact on the health of the nation's citizens *and* was able to demonstrate clear quality control on the care provided. The support accrued to nursing over a century could be eroded in a decade if nurses did not learn to state what it was they did for clients, demonstrate that they could do what was described, and provide evidence of the positive effects of the actions taken. A concise universal language of nursing diagnoses could provide a frame for the needed demonstration.

At the same time that practicing nurses (including nurse educators) have been struggling with vocabulary, schools of nursing have continued the perpetual search for teaching materials that are timely, comprehensive, attractive, and a multitude of other adjectives. Textbooks available have often been "not quite right" due to many factors, not the least of which is that each developed a unique language based on the author's understanding of nursing theory, clinical expertise, original school of nursing and publisher. There has seldom been a clear way to measure one book against another for direction given to a practitioner, since terminology about both diagnoses and treatments is inconsistent. A universal taxonomy of diagnoses would stabilize vocabulary so that in comparing books (or articles) one could make more effective choices based on preference for recommended treatments or clarity of presentation about a given condition.

As more nurses have come to describe their professional responsibility as the process of diagnosing and treating client conditions, the amount of work done to clarify diagnostic terminology and to explicate the relationship of diagnoses to theory and practice has multiplied. Fortunately, there has also been a healthy awareness that there is no perfect end-product of this process. Because nursing is a science, the knowledge upon which it is based is continually changing, and the diagnostic language must change as well.

Likewise, more sophisticated nurses will continue to develop more finely subdivided diagnoses and specific treatments, and the language will be further refined. It would be fruitless to "wait until the work is done" before developing textbooks, reference works, and articles for use by practitioners and students. The more nurses who become educated about diagnosing and diagnoses, the richer the scope of work on which to build improvement.

I am delighted, then, to be a small part of such a work: A textbook that acknowledges both the primitive state of our diagnostic vocabulary in nursing and the central role the diagnostic process plays in our practice. I suspect that the responses to the work, by reviewers, nurse educators, and students, will range from gushing delight with a book that is ahead of its time to scornful deprecation of a work too unsophisticated to be useful. Given the range of possible combinations of levels of knowledge about nursing diagnosis and levels of commitment to nursing diagnosis, that is probably appropriate.

All nurses are not at the same place—I believe this text can be put to use by practitioners, especially beginning practitioners, in such a way that the baseline of communication about diagnosing is both more consistent and more advanced than it has been in the past.

Happy and challenging reading!

KRISTINE GEBBIE

Portland, Oregon
1982

PREFACE

Recent years have witnessed the increased attention given to nursing diagnosis by conferences, journal articles, and published texts. Yet, to date, no one volume exists that provides the nursing student and practicing nurse with an overview of information on nursing diagnosis. The purpose of this book is to provide such an overview, one that includes definitions and history of nursing diagnosis, the "how to" of formulating a nursing diagnosis, and the presentation of clinical situations in which nursing diagnoses are developed for clients in a variety of health care settings.

Throughout the text, nursing diagnosis is considered an integral step of the nursing process, even though it is singled out for purposes of examination and clarification. The nursing process model used in the text is a five-step one: assessment, nursing diagnosis, plan, intervention, and evaluation.

The text is divided into three sections: the historical and theoretical development of nursing diagnosis, the realities of utilizing nursing diagnosis, and client models demonstrating the use of nursing diagnoses. Section I discusses the general nature of the diagnostic process and its relevance for the process of nursing diagnosis. In tracing the historical development of nursing process and nursing diagnosis, a variety of definitions of nursing diagnosis are presented, including the definition to be used by this text:

A nursing diagnosis is a statement of a potential or an actual altered health status of a client(s), which is derived from nursing assessment and which requires intervention from the domain of nursing.

This section also examines the relationship of nursing diagnosis to other components within the five-step nursing process model and provides guidelines for the formulation of a nursing diagnosis. Introduced in this section is the topic of *conceptual framework*, specifically that of adaptation. A conceptual framework is relevant to nursing diagnosis, particularly when the diagnostic statements are formulated using a deductive approach.

Section II addresses the benefits and difficulties to the client, nurse, and nursing profession of using nursing diagnoses and discusses the implications diagnosis has for curriculum development and nursing research.

Section III comprises seven chapters, presenting a variety of client examples for whom nursing diagnoses are formulated on the basis of assessment data. The task presented to each of the seven authors was the following: *To illustrate the formulation and utilization of nursing diagnosis within the nursing process in your nursing specialty.* Though each author was given the same task, the strength of the chapters lies in their diversity of style. Authors varied in the number of client situations and nursing diagnoses presented, and nursing care plans are illustrated in a variety of acceptable formats. Some chapters discuss the formulation of diagnoses not only for illness but also health maintenance. Adaptation as a conceptual framework is reflected in varying degrees in the client models. Even with the diversity of style, the consistent belief is expressed that nursing diagnosis is an essential ingredient of the nursing process. In every chapter the nursing diagnostic statement is presented in the context of the five-step nursing process.

Together, these chapters are useful models to study in the search for a realistic, efficient means to utilize nursing diagnosis.

When looking to the future professional role of the nurse, the editors believe in the necessity of the development of a classification system for nursing diagnosis. Such a system has numerous implications for the nursing profession in all areas of education, practice, and research. In the field of education, such a classification system would be incorporated into nursing curricula. Skills would be taught in which the student would analyze assessment data and combine this analysis with nursing knowledge and experience to make a nursing judgment, that is, the formulation of a nursing diagnosis. A classification system of nursing diagnosis would provide a basis for organization of health needs encountered by nurses and would suggest the best way to meet these needs within the domain of nursing. By arranging a hierarchy of nursing diagnoses, a sequential curriculum pattern could be established.

In nursing practice, nursing diagnosis will serve to facilitate the delivery of health care. In the future it is hoped that further refinement and classification of nursing diagnoses will lead to a standard taxonomy by which nurses can identify the therapies that are specific to nursing as well as those that are interdependent and those that are wholly dependent on other health professionals.

In the field of nursing research, the editors feel nursing diagnosis will further identify and describe the domain of nursing as well as further develop nursing knowledge. Nursing diagnosis will facilitate nursing research by identifying nursing problems that can be the basis for research investigations. Findings of such research will contribute to the growth of nursing knowledge.

The editors are well aware that the text's material represents a very beginning effort to understand and articulate the whole of nursing diagnosis. We hope its deficits are offset by the benefits of getting material into the hands of practitioners and students so that they may foster its use and further its development.

This text has occasioned substantial personal and professional growth for the authors and editors. It is hoped that the reader will experience a similar growth. It is further hoped that the nursing diagnosis movement will lead to greater professionalism in nursing and greater utilization of nursing diagnosis in the nursing process by the individual nurse. The ultimate outcome of this endeavor will be greater quality of nursing service to the client.

Acknowledgements

As is true of any major project, many prople have assisted with this endeavor, whose names would not ordinarily appear in print. We gratefully acknowledge the contributions of two indispensable people: Lynne Masterson, who competently and repeatedly typed the manuscript, and Helene Mayhew, who assisted with the typing in the final stages of editing. Last, but most importantly, we thank our families, whose support and tolerance of our "wee hour of the morning" activities enabled us to complete our task.

JUDITH H. CARLSON

CAROL A. CRAFT

ANNE D. MCGUIRE

CONTENTS

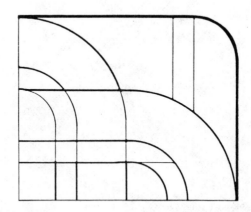

SECTION ONE

NURSING DIAGNOSIS:

Historical and
Theoretical Development

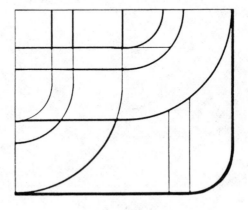

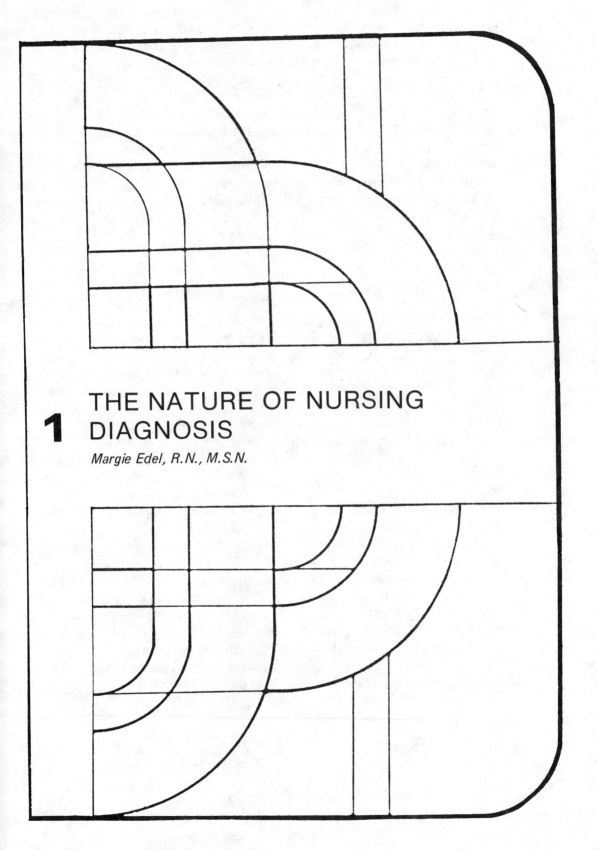

1 THE NATURE OF NURSING DIAGNOSIS

Margie Edel, R.N., M.S.N.

The excitement an architect feels while watching a building take form from his or her design or the excitement parents feel while watching their infant take that first step — such excitement is being generated in nursing today with the development and classification of nursing diagnoses. Although the term nursing diagnosis was proposed many years ago, it is only in the last few years that a great deal of support has been given to accepting and utilizing the term in the practice of nursing. As in many things that are new and in the process of further development, there also exists an element of confusion. *What is a nursing diagnosis? How does it differ from a medical diagnosis? Is there a need for nursing diagnosis? If so, what is the process of diagnosing and what are the competencies necessary to diagnose? What are the potential difficulties and benefits springing from the utilization of nursing diagnoses?* These are but a few of the questions to be considered in this chapter.

WHAT IS A NURSING DIAGNOSIS?

In order to define nursing diagnosis, it is imperative to understand what diagnosis means without the modifier "nursing." Webster (1974) notes that the term, "diagnosis," comes from the Greek word, "diagignoskein," meaning "to distinguish." This in turn was derived from "dia" meaning "through, apart" and from "gignoskein" meaning "to know." Webster further defines diagnosis as "1: the art or act of identifying a disease from its signs and symptoms 2: a concise technical description of a taxon 3a: investigation or analysis of the course or nature of a condition, situation, or problem 3b: a statement or conclusion concerning the nature of some phenomenon." The first component of Webster's definition pertains to diagnoses made by physicians. The second component pertains primarily to the classification of plants and animals, and the third component describes diagnosis as it is used in the profession of nursing.

Anyone who makes a statement or conclusion about the cause or nature of a condition, situation, or problem is by definition diagnosing. Social workers may diagnose economic and social dimensions of their clients. Educators diagnose the nature or cause of a student's inability to learn. Technicians, from the auto mechanic to the aerospace engineer, diagnose the nature or cause of phenomena in their specific field. Nurses diagnose the nature or cause of phenomena requiring nursing care.

A variety of definitions of nursing diagnosis have been formulated in the past 25 years. Those definitions quoted frequently in the current nursing literature appear in Table 1-1.

Table 1-1 Definitions of Nursing Diagnosis

Author of Definition	Definition
Abdellah, 1957	"The determination of the nature and extent of nursing problems presented by the individual patients or families receiving nursing care."
Durand and Prince, 1966	"A statement of a conclusion resulting from a recognition of a pattern derived from a nursing investigation of the patient."
Gebbie and Lavin, 1975	"The judgment or conclusion that occurs as a result of nursing assessment."
Bircher, 1975	"An independent nursing function. . .An evaluation of a client's personal responses to his human experience throughout the life cycle, be they developmental or accidental crises, illness, hardship or other stresses."
Aspinall, 1976	"A process of clinical inference from observed changes in patient's physical or psychological condition; if it is arrived at accurately and intelligently, it will lead to identification of the possible causes of symptomatology."
Gordon, 1976	"Actual or potential health problems which nurses, by virtue of their education and experience, are capable and licensed to treat."

Some of the authors offered further explanation of the terms used within the definition. Abdellah (1957) defined "problem" as "a condition faced by the patient or family that the nurse can assist him or them to meet through the performance of her professional functions."

Bircher (1975) explained that "evaluation of a client's personal response is based on all factors affecting his well-being, dignity, rights, recovery, maintenance, promotion of health, and attainment of a meaningful lifestyle. Thus, a nursing diagnosis includes consideration of the person's needs and concerns in all five realms of human experience and knowledge — the biological, physical-environmental, socio-cultural, psychological, and spiritual-humanistic realms."

Gordon (1976) also clarified what she meant by actual or potential health problems. She stated that those problems would generally include "potential or actual disturbances in life processes, patterns, functions, or development, including those occurring secondary to disease." She described each diagnostic concept or category as having three components. These are (1) the state-of-the-patient, also considered to be the health problem, (2) the etiology of the problem, and (3) signs and symptoms. The first component, state-of-the-patient, is the description of the patient's condition, either actual or potential, for which nursing therapy is given. The second component, etiology, gives direction to the therapy required. The third component, signs and symptoms, provides information necessary to arrive at the diagnosis.

Though the emphasis varies in each of these definitions, there are many similarities. The definitions of Durand and Prince and Gebbie and Lavin are similar because they emphasize that the nursing diagnosis is the result of the nursing assessment. Aspinall also states that the diagnosis results from "observed changes." Other definitions identify the fact that nurses are involved in making judgments. For example, Abdellah points out that nurses make a "determination." Durand and Prince refer to this as "... a conclusion resulting from a recognition of a pattern. ..." Aspinall calls it "clinical inference." Bircher openly states that nursing diagnosis is an independent nursing function, an evaluation.

Also included in some definitions is the entity to be diagnosed. Abdellah describes this entity as the "nursing problems presented by the individual patients or families." Aspinall describes it as a change in the patient's physical or psychological condition. Bircher describes it as the client's responses to human experience. Gordon refers to that which is to be diagnosed as "actual or potential health problems which nurses ... can treat."

For the purpose of this text, the following definition of nursing diagnosis will be used: *A nursing diagnosis is a statement of a potential or actual altered health status of a client(s), which is derived from nursing assessment and which requires intervention from the domain of nursing.* By referring to the entity to be diagnosed as "health status," one avoids the negative connotation of "problem," and allows for positive diagnoses of individuals, families, and communities.

What Are the Differences Between Medical and Nursing Diagnoses?

The differences between medical and nursing diagnoses are reflective of their differing goals. Medical diagnoses focus on pathology, treatment, and cure of disease. Nursing diagnoses focus on the individual's response to illness or other factors that adversely affect, or have the potential to adversely affect, the attainment or maintenance of optimal wellness.

There are instances when diagnoses may be common to several disciplines. For example, the diagnosis of "anxiety" might be made by the nurse, the social worker, or the physician, yet both etiology and treatment could differ for each. An individual who had undergone a colon resection and creation of a colostomy for cancer of the colon was diagnosed as anxious by the physician because the patient stated he was extremely upset and had been having nightmares about recurring cancer. The physician prescribed Librium. The social worker diagnosed "anxiety" concerning inability to purchase required colostomy equipment. Her treatment consisted of arranging for financial assistance. The professional nurse diagnosed "anxiety" related to the difficulty the patient was having in caring for the colostomy. The treatment by the nurse consisted of teaching the patient colostomy care to achieve optimal control.

In some instances, particularly emergency situations, the nursing diagnosis and medical diagnosis may be the same initially and then change after initial therapeutic actions have been taken. For instance, respiratory arrest could be appropriately diagnosed by both physicians and nurses and would require immediate ventilation. Following that intervention, the medical diagnosis might become "myasthenic crisis," and the nursing diagnosis, "severe anxiety related to intubation."

A nursing diagnosis may also be indicative of a medical diagnosis and vice versa. A nursing diagnosis of "severe chest pain" might be indicative of the medical diagnosis, "myocardial infarction." Similarly, a medical diagnosis of "quadraplegia" might be indicative of the nursing diagnosis, "potential alteration of skin integrity."

Thus it can be seen that medical and nursing diagnoses differ in as much as medicine and nursing differ and are similar in as much as medicine and nursing are similar. As nursing and medicine collaborate and strive toward the betterment of the overall health status of the client(s), their diagnoses also overlap and complement each other.

Is There a Need for Nursing Diagnoses?

"Need" refers to an urgent requirement for something essential or desirable that is lacking. In order to answer the question as presented, it must be determined if there is indeed something essential or desirable in the nursing process that is lacking. It is now generally accepted that professional nurses do offer independent nursing therapies that have a scientific base. These therapies are referred to in the nursing process as "interventions." If the nursing process is considered complete without a nursing diagnosis, then those interventions would be planned immediately following the nursing assessment. The nursing assessment, an important and basic step in the nursing process, would lack conclusions or findings. Without nursing diagnoses, there would be no specific identification of the health problem(s) or status for which nursing care is initiated.

It is inconceivable that planning would be appropriate or logical if the total assessment data were not analyzed and the alterations not identified. It seems essential that if the professional nurse is independently offering therapies for "something," that the "something" must first be identified. The identification of that "something" is the diagnosis. Also, if the nursing process is scientifically based, the classification of diagnoses would be feasible, thus offering a universal description of the entire domain of nursing. Through the classification and utilization of nursing diagnoses, the independent functions of nursing can be made clear and specific alterations of health status as identified from analysis of assessment data can be stated.

What Are the Benefits Derived from Nursing Diagnoses?

In addition to strengthening the nursing process through the identification of alterations specified in the assessment data, there are many other benefits derived from the use of nursing diagnosis (Table 1–2). Nursing diagnoses offer an efficient form of communication, specific direction for nursing intervention, standardized organization and structure for education and research, and effective avenues for establishing accountability.

Table 1–2 Benefits Derived from Nursing Diagnoses

Provide efficiency, clarification, and standardization.	A diagnosis is a "shorthand" form of communication which imparts a great deal of information and allows for efficiency, clarification, and standardization. This in turn provides a common discourse; encourages collaboration for clinicians, educators, students, and researchers; and serves as a basis for continuity of care.
Provide purpose and direction.	Nursing therapies as well as signs and symptoms are specific to each diagnosis. Therefore, diagnoses provide purpose and direction for nursing process.
Facilitate research and education.	The development and classification of nursing diagnoses is accomplished through research. Once developed, the classification of diagnoses will provide the organization, structure, and common base from which further research could be conducted, and around which educational programs could be planned. In this way, nursing diagnoses would contribute to the expansion of nursing's unique body of knowledge.
Delineate independent nursing function	Nursing diagnoses would assist in formulating standards, thus clarifying and delineating independent functions of the nursing profession to the public, third-party payers, and all others concerned.
Increase accountability	The individual nurse making a diagnosis would be held accountable for that diagnosis. Such accountability would serve as a stimulus for the individual nurse to expand her knowledge, sharpen data-gathering skills, increase the depth of self-understanding and sensitivity to human needs, and increase an awareness of the issues affecting nursing and health care.

Efficient Form of Communication

Nursing diagnoses would speed communication. Without diagnoses, one nurse would have to relate all of the pertinent assessment factors to another nurse in order to transmit the information needed. That same information could be communicated through diagnoses, for each diagnosis would contain assessment parameters, that is, signs and symptoms specific to each (Fig. 1–1). For example, if a nurse reports to another that Mr. Smith has Diagnosis I, it is immediately known what problem is being referred to, including the specific signs and symptoms. Such communication would also facilitate teaching, consultation, and comparison.

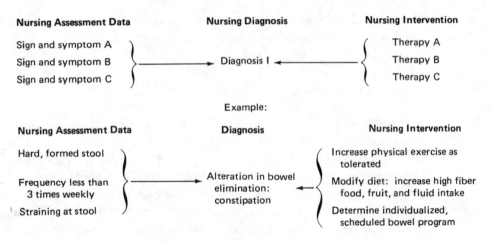

Figure 1-1 Information Specific to Diagnoses

Specific Direction for Intervention

A frame of reference and direction for nursing intervention is lacking when diagnoses are not included in the total nursing process. Not only are signs and symptoms specific to each diagnosis, but intervention are diagnosis-specific too (see Fig. 1–1). Without diagnoses, each individual nurse initiates a "hit or miss" approach to nursing intervention. Nursing literature emphasizes the importance of evaluating the effects of nursing interventions, and if the effects are undesirable or ineffective, the nurse tries another approach. A diagnosis would focus evaluation back through the entire nursing process and would consider the possibility of an error in the diagnosis or a missed diagnosis, rather than focusing only on the nursing therapy. The diagnosis would provide a frame of reference from which one could determine (1) what to do and (2) what to expect. Thus, through the use of nursing diagnoses, a great deal of information becomes synthesized into concise statements, and it becomes possible to bear abstract knowledge on specific phenomena.

Organization and Structure for Research and Education

Jacox (1974) stated that the first step of theory development is "a period of specifying, defining, and classifying the concepts used in describing the phenomena of the field." The development and classification of nursing diagnoses provide for this first step of theory building in nursing. Efforts to standardize diagnostic labels and determine each label's constellation of signs and symptoms and its implications for treatment stimulate and demand research. Once developed, a taxonomy of nursing diagnoses could provide a focus for clinical nursing research that in turn would provide for the orderly growth of nursing's unique body of knowledge.

The development and classification of nursing diagnoses could also provide organization and structure for nursing education. Nursing diagnoses require that educational programs prepare the student in diagnostic skill development, for example, assessment skills. A taxonomy of nursing diagnoses could also provide educational programs with an orderly, nursing-oriented base for the organization of curriculum content.

Avenue for Accountability in Nursing

A current problem for nursing is the establishment of sophisticated avenues for increasing personal and professional accountability. Although the use of nursing diagnosis is not the only avenue, it does have a great deal to offer toward increasing accountability. When nurses independently offer professional health care to their clients, they alone are responsible for their actions. Accountability implies that those nursing actions (the actual performance) will be judged against some standard of performance. As a profession, those standards of performance must be formulated and applied by professional peers. The use of diagnoses would contribute significantly to this end. Primarily, nursing diagnoses describe and label the content of nursing practice. If certain diagnoses carried with them specific nursing therapies, then those therapies would become the actions to which the nurse would be held accountable. Informing the lay public about the domain of nursing activity as reflected in nursing diagnoses would enhance the consumer's ability to require accountability from nurses. In brief, it would demand and clarify independent function.

One step toward accountability was taken when nursing diagnosis was included in the generic Standards of Nursing Practice developed by the American Nurses' Association. Standard II states:

NURSING DIAGNOSES ARE DERIVED FROM HEALTH STATUS DATA.

Rationale: The health status of the client/patient is the basis for determining the nursing care needs. The data are analyzed and compared to norms when possible.

Assessment Factors:

1. The client's/patient's health status is compared to the norm in order to determine if there is a deviation from the norm and the degree and direction of deviation.
2. The client's/patient's capabilities and limitations are identified.
3. The nursing diagnoses are related to and congruent with the diagnoses of all other professionals caring for the client/patient.

(American Nurses' Association, 1973)

If it can be assumed that legislators are true representatives of the people, then the fact that the term diagnosis is being included in revised nursing practice acts also reflects not only the awareness of the public but also its acceptance of the term. Since 1971, almost all of the states have revised their Nurse Practice Acts to authorize the use of the term diagnosis. Some of the revisions simply removed the prohibitions to diagnosis and treatment, while others articulated the nursing role in greater detail and included diagnosing in a broader scope of functioning.

The use of diagnoses would also increase each individual nurse's personal accountability. It would require that each professional nurse become more discriminating and purposeful in gathering and analyzing assessment data and making scientifically based judgments that culminate in the statement of the diagnosis. For when one diagnoses, one becomes vulnerable; the responsibility for the diagnosis rests on that individual making the diagnosis. This in turn would require the nurse to maintain a current, thorough knowledge base and would stimulate an awareness of the current changes in the health care system — especially legal issues originating from the identification of nursing diagnoses and independent nursing function.

WHAT IS THE PROCESS OF DIAGNOSING?

What sequence of intellectual activities is involved in arriving at a diagnosis? This is not an easy question to answer, since this is an abstract process that varies greatly from one individual to another. Literature of other professions as well as nursing is helpful in understanding the possible sequences of these mental activities.

Morgan and Engel (1969) state that the diagnostic process involves a systematic analysis of signs and symptoms and related data. Following the data collection, one must first decide which findings are abnormal by comparing them to accepted standards and to the individual's previous status. The next steps are to locate the abnormal findings and interpret them in terms of underlying morphological, biochemical, physiological, microbiological, or psychosocial factors. The etiology and classification systems are continuously considered. Finally, the personal experience of the patient is evaluated in order to gain an understanding of his illness (Table 1–3). Thus Morgan and Engel view the diagnostic process as involving six separate but interrelated steps.

Table 1–3 Morgan and Engel Diagnostic Process

---

1. Identification of abnormal findings
2. Location of abnormal findings
3. Interpretation of abnormal findings
4. Consideration of etiology
5. Classification
6. Evaluation of effect on individual patient

Judge and Zuidema (1963) have identified the elements of diagnostic logic as a sequence of six events (Table 1–4). Decisions are made at each step of the sequence. *Observation* includes gathering the data. At this point, one decides what is normal and what is abnormal, and the severity is graded. The *description* involves tabulating the observations; irrelevant material is eliminated; relevant findings are condensed and concentrated into usable form, and these findings are systematized into logical clusters or patterns. The decision to be made in this step concerns what is pertinent and what is not. *Interpretation* involves comparing the tabulated data with a known body of knowledge. The decision made here concerns the degree of correspondence between the findings in the patient and the patterns described in the known classification system. *Verification* involves a plan or course of action that includes suitable studies and diagnostic procedures. The decision in this step concerns selecting the proper tests, determining their priority, and interpreting their results. Diagnosis involves applying the final label, the *decision.* At this point, one determines which label most accurately fits. *Action* involves determining a course based on the diagnosis. The decision here is selecting the proper treatment.

Table 1–4   Judge and Zuidema Diagnostic Process

1. Observe
2. Describe
3. Interpret
4. Verify
5. Decide
6. Act

Although the processes just described are systematic, there are differences. Whereas the process described by Morgan and Engel is not entirely sequential, that of Judge and Zuidema is. Morgan and Engel consider the individual's response, which allows for differences. Judge and Zuidema do not include this as a separate step. Whereas Morgan and Engel emphasize pathology, the process of Judge and Zuidema is general and non-specific to the medical profession.

Educators view the diagnostic process as a dynamic process highlighted by flexibility (Kaufman and Kaufman, 1977 and Waugh and Bush, 1971). Kaufman and Kaufman (1977) state that the diagnostic process begins with a "thorough and comprehensive approach to assessment," which requires a thorough repertoire of instruments. Next, he states that one integrates the students' patterns of strengths and weaknesses with characteristic behaviors and then makes comparisons from a variety of normative samples. One then determines when behaviors reach abnormal proportions. Such a determination requires experience and a thorough understanding of the child, developmentally and clinically, and is based on knowledge and intuitive understanding. Then this is translated into practical suggestions for remediation. This process is represented in Table 1–5.

Table 1-5   Kaufman and Kaufman Diagnostic Process

1. Assess thoroughly and comprehensively
2. Integrate strengths and weaknesses
3. Make comparisons
4. Determine abnormal behaviors
5. Make suggestions for remediation

Another author, Andrea Bircher, has made a significant contribution to the understanding of nursing diagnosis through the delineation of the steps of the process of diagnosing. Bircher (1975) divides the process into ten steps that include the development of a taxonomy (Table 1–6). It is Bircher's belief that the first five steps are being accomplished daily by professional nurses and the remainder are in stages of development. This is true for the nursing profession as a whole. It is essential that a common, workable taxonomy of nursing diagnoses be developed and agreed upon by members of the profession if maximum benefits are to be derived from its use. But until the universal taxonomy is developed, the individual professional nurse must diagnose by selecting her own organizing principle and developing her own working taxonomy.

Table 1-6   Bircher Diagnostic Process

1. Noticing
2. Describing
3. Labeling
4. Grouping
5. Identifying significant relationships
6. Noting critical attributes
7. Selecting an organizing principle
8. Developing criteria
9. Developing a taxonomy
10. Diagnosing

Bircher (1975) maintains that there are specific competencies necessary to complete each step of the process. "Noticing" requires that one observes systematically and recognizes significant phenomena. "Describing" requires the ability to give a descriptive narrative verbally and in writing. "Labeling" requires the identification of common elements and patterns, concept formation, and inferential reasoning. "Grouping," Bircher continues, requires coding and identifying factors "to arrange, order, or rate a number of phenomena according to shared characteristics or qualities and their constellations." "Identifying significant relationships" requires the ability to identify values, purpose, relevance, and significance. "Noting critical attributes" requires concisely describing the categories that have at least one significant attribute in common. This step, Bircher states, is being addressed by the National Conference on Classification of Nursing Diagnosis. "Selecting an organizing principle" requires inductive and deductive reasoning and development of first-level theory in order to discretely categorize. "Developing criteria" requires deductive logic, definition, and instrumental reasoning in order to identify the specific criteria and their patterns that must be present in order to assign a given category of a classification system. "Developing a taxonomy," Bircher explains, requires that a conceptual framework be developed and utilized to describe the categories and the nature of their relationships. And lastly, "diagnosing" requires clinical inference that allows one "to identify a new phenomenon; to ascertain the nature, characteristics, origin, and cause of this new phenomenon; to determine its equivalence with one of the categories of a taxonomic classification system; and to assign the new phenomenon to the appropriate category by labeling it with the name of the category."

Comparisons of the diagnostic process as viewed by these authors reveal similarities and differences. All of them stress the steps of identification of special phenomena and interpreting that phenomena to arrive at a diagnosis. They differ in the fact that all of the authors, with the exception of Bircher, assume and depend on a pre-existing taxonomy or classification system; Bircher does not mention this because no such taxonomy exists in nursing at the present time. Until a universal taxonomy for nursing is established, individual professional nurses will formulate and utilize their own classification systems and diagnoses. The step of diagnosing will definitely become more specific and accurate as the taxonomy of nursing diagnosis is further refined.

Through comparison of the various approaches to the diagnostic process, it can be seen that there are certain competencies the professional nurse must possess in order to carry out this process (Fig. 1-2). To make a diagnosis, the nurse must be competent in data-gathering strategies. All assessment data must be identified for correct pattern recognition. The nurse must also possess a strong background of theoretical knowledge in order to distinguish relevant data and group phenomena, and to interpret correctly. The diagnostician must know the signs, symptoms, and relationships that characterize the various categories. Because nursing does not have a standardized taxonomy, this competency is influenced greatly by the examples seen in the practice setting, and by the individual nurse's philosophy and conceptual framework. Another requirement of the diagnostician that is very difficult to teach is that of intuition. This is part of the "art" of nursing, the exercise of recognition, the "flash of light." It is the intuitive judgment that is not subject to the usual rules of logic. At some point in the study of the assessment data, there must be recognition that a particular example does have the qualities that characterize a particular category. The nurse therefore must possess certain skills, knowledge, and intuitive recognition in order to diagnose.

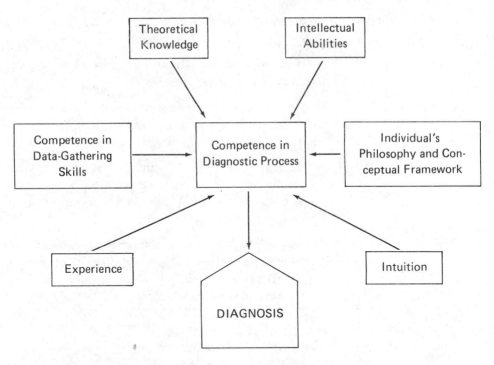

Figure 1-2   Factors Affecting Ability to Diagnose

WHAT ARE THE DIFFICULTIES RELATED TO THE USE OF DIAGNOSES?

Even when diagnoses are made by the most competent diagnostician, there are actual and potential difficulties with which everyone involved must be aware. These difficulties are common to all diagnoses and are not specific to nursing. Table 1–7 gives a brief description of some of these difficulties.

Table 1–7   Difficulties Related to Nursing Diagnoses

Lack of Uniformity	Difference in precision of terms: Results from fact that classification is a dynamic process and is continuously changing. What one nurse might call "alteration in self-concept," another might label "alteration in body image."
Incomplete Development and Vagueness	Lack of sufficient knowledge prohibits formulation of complete, clear, specific definitions. Leads to lack of agreement among those making the diagnoses. A classic example is found in medicine: "Dropsy" was accepted as a diagnosis until new knowledge permitted more refined diagnoses to take its place.
Variations in Severity	The diagnoses for two different individuals may be the same (example: "alterations in skin integrity"), but because of the difference in severity, the constellation of signs and symptoms and the treatment may vary.

Table 1-7 Difficulties Related to Nursing Diagnoses *(Continued)*

Incorrect or Missed Diagnoses	Either a wrong diagnosis is made or a diagnosis that should have been made was not identified. Results from errors or omissions in assessment or in misinterpretation of the data.
Premature Diagnoses	Diagnosis is made before all assessment data is available. For example, a diagnosis of "grief — stage of denial" might be made before it could be determined if the patient had been told of his poor prognosis.
Threat to Individualized Care	A diagnosis implies a certain constellation of signs and symptoms and nursing therapies. The threat exists, therefore, that if a diagnosis is made, therapies are automatically carried out without regard for the individuality of the patient.
Stereotyping	The diagnosis becomes a brand that remains regardless of what current assessment data indicate. For example, diagnosis of "non-compliant" made in the past remains associated with a patient even though his behavior now does not indicate such.

Bircher (1975) responded to the problems of diagnosis by stating that "the values or detriments of diagnosis are not inherent in diagnosis itself, but are a function of the cognitive adequacy or cognitive insufficiency of the user of the tool of diagnosis." These problems or dangers of diagnosing can be avoided by continual systematic, thorough re-assessment of the individual's needs and resources with frequent updating of the diagnoses and individualization of care. It must be remembered that the diagnosis is not an end in itself, and the benefits derived from the development and utilization of nursing diagnoses in the practice of nursing are numerous and far outweigh the actual or potential difficulties.

SUMMARY

The definition of the term diagnosis has made it clear that the term involves activities that are not unique to any group or profession, and that its true meaning is derived from the addition of a modifier such as nursing. A nursing diagnosis, therefore, is defined in this text as *"a statement of a potential or actual altered health status of a client(s), which is derived from nursing assessment and which requires intervention from the domain of nursing."*

The needs for nursing diagnoses are many, but they may all be embodied in one need — the need for survival. For if nursing does have independent functions, then must we not identify them through the use of nursing diagnoses? Any obstacle placed in the way of the continued development and classification of nursing diagnoses endangers the profession itself.

The steps involved in the process of diagnosing are viewed somewhat differently by various authors, but there is agreement that it is an art and a science involving both scientific logic and intuition and that certain competencies are required of the individual making the diagnosis.

There are problems and dangers that may result from the use of diagnoses but they are not inevitable. They can be avoided by continual systematic evaluation and re-assessment, frequent updating of the diagnoses, and individualization of care.

The beneficial effects resulting from the use of diagnoses far outweigh the problems. Nursing diagnoses would give purpose and direction to therapeutic actions and facilitate communication and collaboration in practice, education, and research. Nursing diagnoses would contribute to nursing's unique body of knowledge and articulate the realm of nursing to others. Accountability of the profession and the individual nurse would be increased. Nursing diagnoses would encourage and promote individual growth of the professional nurse and enhance continuity of nursing care. In short, the development and utilization of nursing diagnoses would clarify and demand the independent functions of nursing.

References

Abdellah, F.G.: Method of identifying covert aspects of nursing problems. *Nursing Research, 57:4*, 1957.

American Nurses' Association: *Standards of Nursing Practice.* Kansas City, Mo., American Nurses' Association, 1973.

Aspinall, M.J.: Nursing diagnosis — The weak link. *Nursing Outlook 24:*433, 1976.

Bircher, A.: On the development and classification of diagnoses. *Nursing Forum, 14:*10, 1975.

Durand, M. and Prince, R.: Nursing diagnosis: Process and decision. *Nursing Forum, 5:*50, 1966.

Gebbie, K.M., and Lavin, M.A. (eds.): *Classification of Nursing Diagnoses — Proceedings of the First National Conference.* St. Louis, The C.V. Mosby Company, 1975.

Gordon, M.: Nursing diagnosis and the diagnostic process. *American Journal of Nursing, 76:*1298, 1976.

Jacox, A.: Theory construction in nursing: An overview. *Nursing Research, 23:4*, 1974.

Judge, R., and Zuidema, G.: (eds.): *Physical Diagnosis: A Physiologic Approach to the Clinical Examination,* 2nd ed. Boston, Little, Brown and Company, 1963.

Kaufman, A. and Kaufman, N.: *Clinical Evaluation of Young Children with the McCarthy Scales.* New York, Grune and Stratton, 1977.

Morgan, W., and Engel, G.: *The Clinical Approach to the Patient.* Philadelphia, W.B. Saunders Company, 1969.

Waugh, K., and Bush, W.J.: *Diagnosing Learning Disorders.* Columbus, Ohio, Charles E. Merrill Publishing Company, 1971.

Webster's New Collegiate Dictionary. Springfield, Ma., G. & C. Merriam Company, 1974.

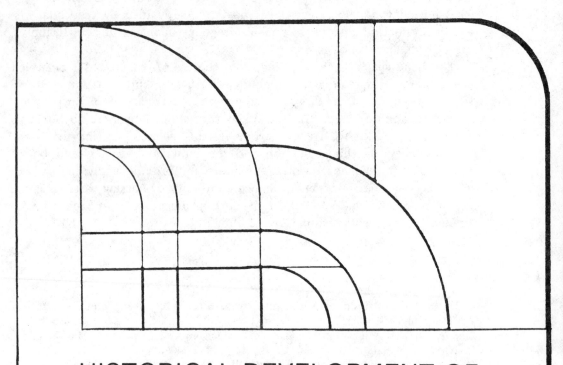

2 HISTORICAL DEVELOPMENT OF NURSING DIAGNOSIS

Florence K. Stelzer, R.N., M.S.N.
Ann Marie Becker, R.N., M.S.N.

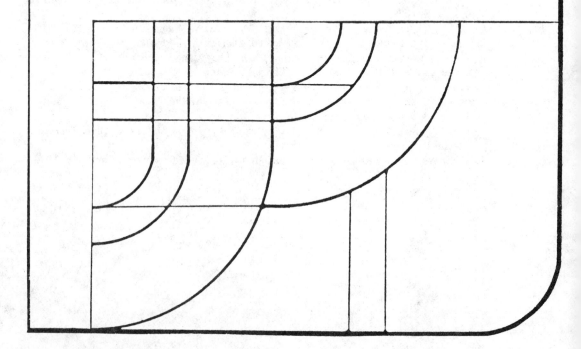

The term nursing diagnosis has gradually become accepted and utilized within the nursing profession; it is a distinct entity within the nursing process, the foundation of a classification system for the nursing profession, and a vital component of education, practice, and research in the field of nursing. This chapter highlights the growth of nursing diagnosis by presenting a brief history of the nursing process and use of the term nursing diagnosis.

EVOLUTION OF THE NURSING PROCESS

The history of the nursing process can be divided into two main phases, the phase of initiation and the phase of identification and analysis. During the phase of initiation, which spanned the years 1850 to 1950, nurses made their initial efforts to structure the process of delivering quality nursing care. The phase of identification and analysis, 1955 to the present, represents the attempts by authors to identify and analyze the nursing process by dividing it into separate steps or components.

The Phase of Initiation

Ever since nursing was first practiced, nurses have engaged in a process to identify health related problems and initiate nursing actions to resolve them. In 1859, Florence Nightingale attempted to add more structure to this process when she emphasized the importance of observation in her *Notes on Nursing*: "The most important practical lesson that can be given to nurses is to teach them what to observe; how to observe — what symptoms indicate improvement — what the reverse — which are of importance — which are of none — which are the evidence of neglect — and of what kind of neglect." Today, observation remains a primary factor in the first step of the nursing process, assessment.

During the first several decades of the 1900's, nursing leaders were incorporating into nursing the investigative methods used by peers in other fields of science and general education. One of these methods, problem-solving, was used by nurses through a case study approach. The case study report described in Deborah MacLurg Jensen's, *Students Handbook on Nursing* (1929) was started at Yale University School of Nursing and was the principal means by which students were being prepared for public health nursing. The studies included an analysis of why the patient came to the hospital, what he would do after hospitalization, and how the nurse could help him (Henderson, 1973). These questions prefigure three of today's components of the nursing process: assessment, plan, and intervention.

By the time Esther Lucille Brown's study *Nursing for the Future*, or the "Brown Report," was published in 1948, most nursing students had become familiar with problem-solving methods such as the case study and written care plans. The "Brown Report" was a major impetus for nursing growth.

The following are three of its main recommendations:

- Schools of nursing should be affiliated with universities
- The term "professional nurse" should be used only for graduates of accredited professional schools
- Adequate remuneration should be made for the professional services of the nurse

The belief that the professional nurse should be academically educated and receive adequate remuneration for services implied that the nurse should be accountable for quality nursing care. At this time there were no adequate means to evaluate the professional nurse's accountability for quality nursing care. This lack was yet another impetus for nurses to identify more clearly the function of nursing. The phase of initiation, which is illustrated in Table 2–1, set the stage for the identification and analysis of the nursing process.

Table 2–1 Initiation Phase of the Nursing Process

Year			
1948			Urgent need to verify quality of nursing care performed.
1929		Nursing Case Studies Analyze: (1) Why patient came to hospital. (2) What patient would do at home. (3) How the nurse can help.	
1859	Vital importance of observation.		
	Nightingale	Jensen	Brown

Phase of Identification and Analysis

It was not until 1955 that Lydia Hall formally described nursing as a process (Hall, 1955). With impetus from Hall's statement, nurses began to analyze the process by its division into steps. Although such a division is an artificial exercise, it is useful in analyzing the nursing process.

Dorothy Johnson (1959), Ida Orlando (1961), and Ernestine Wiedenbach (1963) were some of the first to devise methods to study and identify the steps of the nursing process. They each devised a different three-step process as illustrated in Table 2–2.

Table 2–2 Identification of the Nursing Process: Three Steps

1959 D. Johnson	1961 I. Orlando	1963 E. Wiedenbach
The process of analyzing nursing problems:	Elements in the deliberative action of the nurse:	Steps taken by the nurse to meet the requests of the patients:
1. Assessment	1. Behavior of patient	
2. Decision	2. Reaction of nurse	1. Identify need for help
3. Action	3. Nursing actions designed for the benefit of the patient.	2. Ministration of help
		3. Validation if help given was help needed

In the latter part of the 1960's there was much progress in attempts by the nursing profession to define the process of nursing with more specific terminology. In 1967, Lois Knowles presented a new approach to describing the nursing process. She described successful nursing care as the involvement of five actions or "five D's": discover, delve, decide, do, and discriminate. Though interesting and valid, this approach to nursing was not widely used by the profession.

In 1967, The Western Interstate Commission on Higher Education (WICHE) met to discuss curricular content for graduate nursing programs. During their deliberations they defined nursing process as "that which goes on between a patient and a nurse in a given setting; it incorporates the behaviors of patient and nurse and the resulting interaction." They then identified five steps expressive of the cognitive use of the nursing process: (1) perception, (2) communication, (3) interpretation, (4) intervention, and (5) evaluation.

Also in 1967, a faculty group at the School of Nursing at Catholic University of America identified four phases of the nursing process, which were described in *The Nursing Process*, a text by Helen Yura and Mary Walsh (1967). Dolores Little and Doris Carnevali, writing about nursing care plans, utilized four similar phases of nursing care planning (1969). Interestingly, both groups of authors defined their first phase as including the *observation or health assessment and statement or designation of the problem.*

Most nursing educators continued to view assessment with the inclusion of the problem or diagnosis until Doris Bloch (1974) pointed out the incongruency of the two in an article discussing the overlap of nursing terms and the need to clarify them. She noted that the term assessment as used at that time in nursing was not clearly and consistently defined. She argued that it embodied two conceptually distinct processes: assessment and nursing diagnosis. She suggested a slightly revised five-step model of the nursing process that was compatible with the four-step nursing process. Bloch preferred the terms assessment and nursing diagnosis but chose to use data collection and problem definition because of the clarity of the terms and their "fit" with the problem-oriented record. However, other nursing authors such as Roy (1975b), Mundinger and Jauron (1975), Aspinall (1976), and

Sundeen and coworkers (1976) advocated the use of the term nursing diagnosis and began to use the five-step nursing process. Today, the five-step process has become accepted and utilized by many nurse practitioners, educators, and researchers. Table 2–3 illustrates the evolution of the nursing process from four to five steps.

Table 2–3 Evolution of Nursing Process from Four to Five Steps

1967 H. Yura and M. Walsh	1969 D. Little and D. Carnevali	1974 D. Bloch	1975 Sr. C. Roy	1975 M. Mundinger and G. Jauron
Assessing	Observation	Collection of data Definition of problem	Collection of data	Data gathering
			Nursing diagnosis	**Diagnosing**
Planning	Goals	Planning	Plan for nursing action	Planning
Implementing	Nursing action	Implementation of interventions	Implementation	Implementing
Evaluation	Evaluation	Evaluation	Evaluation	Evaluating

EVOLUTION OF NURSING DIAGNOSIS

As previously mentioned, the nursing profession has always sought to identify patient problems. Perhaps the earliest attempt to publish common problems nurses encountered with patients was by Florence Wilson (1929a, b, c), who wrote a series of three articles analyzing problems experienced by nursing students while caring for patients. Wilson, a nurse educator, modified the case study report outline by inserting the question, "What difficulties did you encounter in nursing this patient?" As illustrated in Figure 2–1, the content of the case study used by nurses over fifty years ago is amazingly similar to assessment forms of today. Wilson's students identified problems reflective of present nursing diagnoses — loneliness, fear, hopelessness, fluid balance, nutrition, and skin integrity.

The term nursing diagnosis was introduced long before it was accepted as a separate component of the process. Five years before Lydia Hall (1955) declared that "nursing is a process," R. Louise McManus (1950) used the term diagnosis in reference to identification of nursing problems when discussing the functions of the professional nurse. Several years later, Vera Fry (1953) boldly used the term nursing diagnosis. Fry was the first to suggest a means of formulating a nursing diagnosis. She advocated observation of five areas of patient needs on which to base a nursing diagnosis: (1) treatment and medication, (2) personal hygiene, (3) environmental needs, (4) guidance and teaching, and (5) human or self needs. Fry stated

Case Study Outline

Patient's name
    Date of admission
    Diagnosis
I.   Relevant Information
    1. Social history
        a. Age
        b. Occupation
        c. Number dependents
        d. Points in personality that you can use in gaining cooperation
    2. Medical history
        a. Dispensary or other past history
        b. Present illness (up to the time you start taking care of the patient)
        c. Laboratory findings and their significance
        d. Physical findings relative to this disease
II.   Problems of Nursing Care
    1. Symptoms
        a. The symptoms should include:
            (1) Any change in cardinal symptoms, such as increase in pulse rate or change in the quality of the pulse or respiration
            (2) Any abnormal conditions that you observe, such as eruption on the skin, jaundice, or cyanosis
            (3) Any abnormal condition of which the patient tells you, such as pain located in the pit of the stomach
        b. Underline those symptoms that you associate with the diagnosis
    2. Nursing treatments, results
    3. Medication, results
    4. Treatments and tests by the doctor with which the nurse assists
    5. Progress
    6. What difficulties were encountered in nursing this patient? Give any attempted solutions.
    7. What did you enjoy about nursing this patient?
    8. What questions do you have about this case?
III.   Plans for this Patient
    1. What medical future does this patient look forward to?
    2. What instruction was the patient given on his discharge for his care at home?
    3. What are the social adjustments and plans for the patient?
IV.   References Read on this Disease

Figure 2-1 Case study outline used by Wilson in 1929

that "once the patient's needs have been identified, we go on to the next step in making the nursing diagnosis . . . the synthesis of each of the first four needs with the human or self needs" (Fry, 1953). Fry challenged nurses to individualize care by using information specific to the individual patient.

Following these developments, various authors began to justify the use of diagnosis by nurses. Lesnick and Anderson (1955) pointed out the legal accountability of the nurse when using professional knowledge to make decisions in giving care. They state: ". . . there is an area with which the nurse is charged, and that area may well be called 'nursing diagnosis.' " Gertrude Hornung (1956) advocated adoption of nursing diagnosis terminology to be used in the work of professional nurses. She said: ". . . vague descriptions of the patient's condition would disappear from our vocabulary." Dorothy Johnson (1959), Faye Abdellah (1960), and Wilda Chambers (1962) are but a few who wrote about nursing diagnosis as an independent function of the professional nurse.

During the 1950s and 1960s there was continuous debate and confusion over use of the term diagnosis and its implied medical connotation. Because of this the terms *problem* or *need* were still more prevalent. Myra Levine (1965) attempted to skirt the entire issue by suggesting an alternative term, *trophicognosis*, which incorporated the concepts of the nurses' observations and the process of cognitive decisions. However, this was not accepted by members of the nursing profession, who chose to continue with the terms *need*, *problem*, or *diagnosis* with the hope that one acceptable term would eventually emerge. Despite the controversy over terminology, there was an increasing contingency of authors who continued to use the term diagnosis (Durand and Prince, 1966; Rothberg, 1967). The increasing awareness of nursing diagnosis in the 1960s was the impetus for a multidisciplinary group to begin research concerning nursing diagnosis (Kelly, 1964; 1966; Hammond, 1966; Hammond, Kelly, Schneider, and Vancini, 1966). Their studies of the diagnostic or inferential process by the nurse have set the groundwork for future research of this complex task.

The seventies brought the expansion of nursing diagnosis and the need for a system of organization of diagnoses to many nurses and other health professionals. The continuing development of this concept was influenced by several factors:

- The inclusion of nursing diagnosis as a responsibility of the nurse in Nurse Practice Acts and Standards of Practice
- The increasing use of the term as noted in the literature of the seventies
- The need for a classification system for nursing diagnosis
- The convening of National Conferences on the Classification of Nursing Diagnoses

An indication of the status of nursing diagnosis within the profession of nursing in the seventies can be found by examining revised nurse practice acts. By 1975, 21 states had revised their nurse practice acts to provide for expanded roles for registered nurses. Fifteen other nurse practice acts were identified that did not prohibit diagnosis and treatment (Bullough, 1975). With the inclusion of nursing diagnosis as a function of the professional nurse in nurse practice acts and with the realization of their legal responsibilities, nurses began to make more use of diagnoses in their nursing activities.

Another major factor in the acceptance of nursing diagnosis by the profession was its inclusion in the Standards of Nursing Practice (1973) developed to provide a basis for measuring the quality of nursing practice.

Standard II states: "Nursing diagnoses are derived from health status data" (Standards of Nursing Practice, 1973). This standard makes nursing diagnosis an integral part of a process whose purpose is to provide high quality nursing care. Nursing specialty organizations have also developed similar standards of practice for use by their members. With the development of these standards, the responsibility of the nurse to diagnose is again identified.

This formal recognition of nursing diagnosis can be attributed to all the previously mentioned efforts by nursing professionals. Nursing literature in the early seventies also reflects the profession's respect for the term diagnosis as well as the justification to begin utilizing nursing diagnosis. As early as 1970, an assessment tool and resultant data were used to formulate a nursing diagnosis (Hamdi and Hutelmeyer, 1970). By 1972 nurses were making nursing diagnoses and subsequently writing nursing orders in one midwest health care institution (Carlson, 1972).

The literature of the mid-seventies demonstrates the effect of the revised Nurse Practice Acts, Standards of Practice, and other activities related to nursing diagnosis. It was not until the formal recognition of the term nursing diagnosis that it was incorporated as a distinct step in the nursing process, as advocated by Bloch (1974), Roy (1975b), Aspinall (1976), and others. The utilization of nursing diagnosis in clinical practice was also addressed more frequently. Mundinger and Jauron (1975) reported on experiences with assisting primary nurses to develop nursing diagnoses that were meaningful and effective in their clinical setting. Roy (1975b), in a presentation to the AORN members, provided an example of an operating room nurse of the future and her use of nursing diagnoses within the nursing process. In the area of research, Goodwin and Edwards (1975) discussed the use of a computer program devised to collect data and formulate nursing diagnoses.

Despite the increased utilization of nursing diagnoses in the early seventies, there was not much collaboration or systemized use of nursing diagnoses among nurses throughout the country. Faculty members at St. Louis University School of Nursing and Allied Health Professions identified the need for more formalized activities in the development and classification of nursing diagnostic labels. This need led them to schedule the first National Conference on Classification of Nursing Diagnoses, which was held in 1973.

During the mid-seventies there was continued discussion about the necessity for developing a classification system. The following advantages of a classification system have been noted by Gebbie and Lavin (1974), Brown (1974), Bircher (1975), and Roy (1975a):

- Facilitates communication among nurses in education, practice, and research
- Facilitates communication between nurses and others — third party payers, legislators, other government agencies, and the general public
- Provides a systematic description of the phenomena with which nurses are concerned
- Provides a basis for theory development
- Increases the quality of nursing research
- Allows application of epidemiological principles and methods to clinical nursing

This acknowledgement of the need for a classification system was a stimulus for commitment of the nursing profession to future National Conferences on Classification of Nursing Diagnoses.

In any discussion of nursing diagnosis during the seventies, it is important to include an account of the three national conferences that have provided for national and international collaboration among nurses in practice, education, and research. In 1973 the First National Conference on Classification of Nursing Diagnoses was sponsored by St. Louis University School of Nursing and Allied Health Professions. One hundred nurses from across the country participated. The purposes and outcomes of this conference are listed in Table 2-4.

Table 2-4 First National Conference on Classification of Nursing Diagnoses

---

Purposes

1. To begin planning for a classification system for nursing diagnosis.
2. To provide participants with information on the concept of classification systems currently used in medicine and the relationship of a classification system for nursing diagnosis to the health care system.
3. To maintain the commitment of participants to a system of nursing diagnosis.*
4. To disseminate information from the conference.*
5. To test the diagnoses in nursing education, practice, and research.*
6. To explore routes for validation of a classification system by official nursing organizations.*
7. To promote understanding of the concept of nursing diagnosis among other health professionals.*

Outcomes

1. Identification of one hundred nursing diagnoses including characteristics, duration, and etiology.
2. Suggestions by small group participants for inductive approaches to categorize nursing diagnoses.
3. Establishment of a National Group for Classification of Nursing Diagnosis including:
    a. a task force to plan succeeding conferences, promote conferences, promote research, and disseminate information.
    b. a clearinghouse to act as a resource center for information on nursing diagnosis and to publish a newsletter providing information on activities related to nursing diagnosis.
4. Plans for the Clearinghouse to collect data on nursing diagnosis identified by practicing nurses in various nationwide health agencies to be used at the Second National Conference.
5. Publication of proceedings of the conference (Gebbie and Lavin [eds.], 1975).

---

*Long-range goals

The Second National Conference on Classification of Nursing Diagnoses in 1975 was planned by the task force established at the first conference. Some participants from the first conference and other interested nurses, including some from Canada, continued the work begun in 1973 as noted in Table 2-5.

Table 2–5 Second National Conference on Classification of Nursing Diagnoses

Purposes

1. To provide participants with information on major nomenclatures and classification systems being used by health professionals.
2. To review the one hundred diagnoses from the first national conference.
3. To generate and label additional nursing diagnoses (using data collected by the Clearinghouse).

Outcomes

1. Acceptance of 37 diagnoses, including revision of diagnoses from the previous conference with defining characteristics.
2. Listing of nineteen suggested diagnoses to be developed more completely for consideration at the national conference.
3. Suggestions for a possible conceptual framework for nursing diagnosis.
4. Formation of state and regional conference groups to provide for national conference participants and additional interested nurses to:
   a. generate, label, and implement nursing diagnoses and forward their diagnoses to the National Group.
   b. provide local speakers on nursing diagnosis to acquaint interested individuals with the concept.
   c. maintain libraries with an emphasis on holdings related to nursing diagnosis.
5. Publication of a summary of the conference (Gebbie [ed.] , 1976).

A Third National Conference, which was held in 1978, continued the activities of the previous two conferences (Table 2–6). Discussions related to a conceptual framework for nursing diagnosis became more specific at this time. A group of nurse theorists, who believed in the work of the conference but were concerned about an organizing principle, began to develop a conceptual framework, then submitted their recommendations to the conference participants.

Table 2–6 Third National Conference on Classification of Nursing Diagnoses

Purposes

1. To define and refine diagnostic labels using the guidelines for diagnostic categories (Gordon, 1976).
2. To provide an organizing principle for nursing diagnosis.
3. To discuss the use of nursing diagnosis in:
   a. nursing practice
   b. nursing research
   c. nursing administration
   d. nursing education

Table 2–6 Third National Conference on Classification of Nursing Diagnoses *(Continued)*

Outcomes

1. Development or revision of 26 nursing diagnoses with etiology and defining characteristics.
2. Establishment of a speaker's bureau and a list of diagnostic experts who would be available as resource persons for specific diagnostic labels.
3. Recommendations by the theorists' group for:
   a. a conceptual framework of unitary man
   b. a redefinition of nursing diagnosis according to this framework
4. Plans for publication of the conference proceedings.

As the decade of the eighties began, a Fourth National Conference was held to continue and expand on previous activities. This conference differed from the earlier ones in that the agenda provided for specific activities related to the conceptual framework of unitary man, which had been a topic at the third conference.

Table 2–7 Fourth National Conference on Classification of Nursing Diagnoses

Purposes

1. To identify, develop, and refine nursing diagnoses.
2. To review developments in the identification, classification, and utilization of nursing diagnoses in practice, education, and research.
3. To examine a proposed conceptual framework for nursing diagnosis.

Outcomes

1. Formal recognition of 42 nursing diagnoses from previously accepted, new, or revised diagnoses.
2. Continued discussion on the use of unitary man as a conceptual framework for nursing diagnosis.
3. Formation of a committee to develop a more formal organizational structure for the National Group for Classification of Nursing Diagnosis.
4. Plans for publication of the conference proceedings.

In reviewing the long-range goals identified at the first national conference, it can be seen that these goals are being met and that the process begun in 1973 has grown into a national effort. These conferences have indeed provided the opportunity for nurses to collaborate in the processes of classifying and using nursing diagnoses.

The activities of the late seventies demonstrate the influence of nursing diagnoses in the areas of education, practice, and research. During this time, nursing diagnosis was becoming an integral part of nursing education. The utilization of nursing diagnosis as a component of the nursing process was included more frequently in the education of nurses in undergraduate,

graduate, and continuing nursing education programs. Some examples of these activities have been provided by nursing literature, reports by conference participants, and information submitted to the National Clearinghouse for Nursing Diagnosis. They include the following:

- Nursing diagnosis integrated into the conceptual framework of a curriculum
- Nursing diagnosis presented as a distinct part of the nursing process
- Nursing diagnoses providing a framework for nursing content
- Diagnostic process taught to nursing students and utilized in a variety of clinical settings
- Graduate students' seminars held to obtain a consensus on nursing diagnoses
- Continuing education programs offered to provide knowledge about nursing diagnoses to practicing nurses

As more nurses have become educated about nursing diagnoses, they have utilized them in their nursing practice. Some examples of how nursing diagnoses have been implemented in nursing practice during the seventies include the following:

- The term nursing diagnosis used in nursing care plans and kardexes
- Diagnostic statements used as the organizational structure in the formulation of standards and delivery of care
- Consultants and staff development programs to assist nursing staff in identifying nursing diagnoses
- Nursing diagnoses used in discharge and post-discharge planning
- Nursing diagnoses used in primary care
- Nursing diagnoses incorporated into record keeping, reports, and referrals in private practice

Research and its subsequent reporting is of great importance in the identification and classification of nursing diagnoses. Research studies conducted in the late seventies in hopes of generating and validating nursing diagnoses included topics such as:

- Psychophysiological stress in patients with myocardial infarctions
- Maternal attachment
- Digoxin drug incompatibilities
- Post-discharge period
- Powerlessness
- Pain

A description of the activities of the latter seventies would be incomplete if the international interest in nursing diagnosis was not discussed. Canadian nurses have actively participated in the national conferences in the United States and inquiries have been received by the Clearinghouse from Australia, Belgium, Germany, Great Britain, Israel, and Switzerland. In 1977, the First Canadian Conference on Nursing Diagnosis was held in Toronto, Ontario. There has also been some discussion about planning an international conference on nursing diagnosis in the future. In the early seventies there was not much national collaboration on identifying and classifying nursing diagnoses, but now international attention and cooperation are being demonstrated.

SUMMARY

In reviewing the history of professional nursing, one can see the gradual evolution of the nursing process into five steps with nursing diagnosis developing into a distinct step. Today, nursing has accepted nursing diagnosis as an independent function of the professional nurse, one which is *beginning* to be utilized in education, practice, and research. The establishment of a classification system for nursing diagnosis has grown into a national effort. In the future nursing diagnosis will become not only widely utilized by the nursing profession but accepted by other professions and the general public.

References

Abdellah, F.G.: *Patient Centered Approach to Nursing.* New York, Macmillan Company, 1960.

American Nurses' Association: *Standards of nursing practice.* Kansas City, Mo.: American Nurses' Association, 1973.

Aspinall, M.J.: Nursing diagnosis — The weak link. *Nursing Outlook, 24:*433, 1976.

Avant, K.: Nursing diagnosis: Maternal attachment. *Advances in Nursing Science, 2:*45, 1979.

Bircher, A.U.: On the development and classification of diagnoses. *Nursing Forum, 14:*10, 1975.

Bloch, D.: Some crucial terms in nursing — What do they really mean? *Nursing Outlook, 22:*689, 1974.

Brown, E.L.: *Nursing for the Future.* New York, Russell Sage Foundation, 1948.

Brown, M.: The epidemiologic approach to the study of clinical nursing diagnoses. *Nursing Forum, 13:*346, 1974.

Bruce, J.: Implementation of nursing diagnosis. A nursing administrator's perspective. *Nursing Clinics of North America, 14:*509, 1979.

Bullough, B.: The third phase in nursing licensure: The current nurse practice acts. *In* Bullough, B. (ed.): *The Law and the Expanding Nursing Role.* New York, Appleton-Century Crofts, 1975.

Carlson, S.: A practical approach to the nursing process. *American Journal of Nursing, 72:*1589, 1972.

Chambers, W.: Nursing diagnosis. *American Journal of Nursing, 62:* 102, 1962.

Classification of Nursing Diagnoses — Transcripts of the Third National Conference. St. Louis, The Clearinghouse — National Group for Classification of Nursing Diagnoses, 1978.

Classification of Nursing Diagnoses — Transcripts of the Fourth National Conference. St. Louis, The Clearinghouse — National Group for Classification of Nursing Diagnoses, 1980.

Dalton, J.: Nursing diagnosis in a community health setting. *Nursing Clinics of North America, 14:*525, 1979.

Deloughery, G.: *History and Trends of Professional Nursing,* 8th ed. St. Louis, The C.V. Mosby Company, 1977.

Durand, M., and Prince, R.: Nursing diagnosis: Process and decision. *Nursing Forum,* 5:50, 1966.

Feild, L.: The implementation of nursing diagnosis in clinical practice. *Nursing Clinics of North America, 14:*497, 1979.

Fredette, S. and O'Connor, K.: Nursing diagnosis in teaching and curriculum planning. *Nursing Clinics of North America, 14:*541, 1979.

Fry, V.S.: The creative approach to nursing. *American Journal of Nursing, 53:*301, 1953.

Gebbie, K.M. (ed.): *Classification of Nursing Diagnoses — Summary of the Second National Conference.* St. Louis, The Clearinghouse — National Group for Classification of Nursing Diagnoses, 1976.

Gebbie, K., and Lavin, M.A., Classifying nursing diagnoses. *American Journal of Nursing, 74:*250, 1974.

Gebbie, K., and Lavin, M.A., (eds.): *Classification of Nursing Diagnoses — Proceedings of the First National Conference.* St. Louis, The C.V. Mosby Company, 1975.

Goodwin, J.O., and Edwards, B.S.: Developing a computer program to assist the nursing process: Phase 1 — from systems analysis to an expandable program. *Nursing Research, 24:*299, 1975.

Gordon, M.: Nursing diagnoses and the diagnostic process. *American Journal of Nursing, 76:*1298, 1976.

Gordon, M.: The classification of nursing diagnoses. *Journal N.Y. State Nurses' Association, 9:*5, 1978.

Guzzetta, C., and Forsyth, G.L.: Nursing diagnostic pilot study: Psychophysiologic stress. *Advances in Nursing Science, 2:*27, 1979.

Hall, L.E.: Quality of nursing care. *Address at meeting of Department of Baccalaureate and Higher Degree Programs of the New Jersey League for Nursing,* February 7, 1955, Seton Hall University, Newark, N.J. Published in *Public Health News,* New Jersey State Department of Health, June, 1955.

Hamdi, M.E., and Hutelmyer, C.M.: A study of the effectiveness of an assessment tool in the identification of nursing care problems. *Nursing Research, 19:*354, 1970.

Hammond, K.R.: Clinical inference in nursing. A psychologist's viewpoint. *Nursing Research, 15:*27, 1966.

Hammond, R., Kelly, K., Schnieder, R., and Vancini, M.: Clinical inference in nursing. Analyzing cognitive tasks representative of nursing problems. *Nursing Research, 15:*134, 1966.

Henderson, B.: Nursing diagnosis: Theory and practice. *Advances in Nursing Science, 1:*75, 1978.

Henderson, V.: On nursing care plans and their history. *Nursing Outlook, 21:*378, 1973.

Hornung, G.: The nursing diagnosis — An exercise in judgment. *Nursing Outlook, 4:*29, 1956.

Jensen, D.M.: *Student's Handbook on Nursing Case Studies.* New York, Macmillan, 1929.

Johnson, D.: A philosophy of nursing. *Nursing Outlook, 7:*198, 1959.

Jones, P.: A terminology for nursing diagnoses. *Advances in Nursing Science, 2:*65, 1979.

Kelly, K.: An approach to the study of clinical inference in nursing, Part 1. Introduction to the study of clinical inference in nursing. *Nursing Research, 13:*314, 1964.

Kelly, K.: Clinical inference in nursing. A nurse's viewpoint. *Nursing Research, 15:*23, 1966.

Kelly, L.Y.: Nursing practice acts. *American Journal of Nursing, 74:*1310, 1974.

Knowles, L.N.: Decision making in nursing — A necessity for doing. *ANA Clinical Sessions.* New York, Appleton-Century Crofts, 1967, p. 248.

LeSage, J., Beck, C., and Johnson, M.: Nursing diagnosis of drug incompatibility: A conceptual process. *Advances in Nursing Science, 1:*63, 1979.

Lesnik, M., and Anderson, B.: *Nursing Practice and the Law,* 2nd ed. Philadelphia, J.B. Lippincott Company, 1955.

Levine, M. Trophicognosis: An alternative to nursing diagnosis. Exploring progress in medical-surgical nursing practice. *ANA Regional Clinical Conferences, 2:*55, 1965.

Little, D., and Carnevali, D.: *Nursing Care Planning.* Philadelphia, J.B. Lippincott Company, 1969.

McKeehan, K.: Nursing diagnosis in a discharge planning program. *Nursing Clinics of North America, 14*:517, 1979.

McManus, R.L.: Assumptions of the function of nursing. Report of work conference at Plymouth, N.H., June 12–23, 1950. In *Regional Planning for Nursing and Nursing Education.* New York, Bureau of Publications, Teachers' College, Columbia University, 1950, p. 54.

Missouri Nurses' Association Council on Nursing Practice. Explanatory statements, definitions and recommendations — Missouri Revised Statutes, Chapter 335, Sections 011–096. *The Missouri Nurse, 47*:9, 1978.

Mundinger, M., and Jauron, G.: Developing a nursing diagnosis. *Nursing Outlook, 23:*94, 1975.

Nightingale, F.: *Notes on Nursing. What it is, What it is not.* New York, Dover Publications, 1969. (Originally published, 1859.)

Orlando, I. *The Dynamic Nurse-Patient Relationship.* New York, G.P. Putnam's Sons, 1961.

Proceedings of the Canadian Conference on Nursing Diagnosis 1. Toronto, Ontario, University of Toronto, 1978.

Rossi, L., and Haines, V.: Nursing diagnoses related to acute myocardial infarction. *Cardiovascular Nursing, 15*:11, 1979.

Rothberg, J.: Why nursing diagnosis? *American Journal of Nursing, 67*:1040, 1967.

Roy, C.: A diagnostic classification system for nursing. *Nursing Outlook, 23*:90, 1975. (a)

Roy, C.: The impact of nursing diagnosis. *AORN Journal, 21*:1023, 1975. (b)

Roy, C.: Why are we here? Addendum to: Gebbie, K. (ed.): *Classification of Nursing Diagnoses — Summary of the Second National Conference.* St. Louis, The Clearinghouse — National Group for Classification of Nursing Diagnoses, 1976.

Sundeen, S., Stuart, G.W., Rankin, E.D., and Cohen, S.P.: *Nurse-Client Interaction: Implementing the Nursing Process.* St. Louis, The C.V. Mosby Company, 1976.

Weber, S.: Nursing diagnosis in private practice. *Nursing Clinics of North America, 14:*533, 1979.

Western Interstate Commission on Higher Education: Defining clinical content, graduate nursing programs, medical-surgical nursing, Boulder, Colo., 1967.

Wiedenbach, E.: The helping art of nursing. *American Journal of Nursing, 63*:54, 1963.

Wilson, F.: Nursing medical patients: An analysis of problems encountered by student nurses in caring for them. *American Journal of Nursing, 29*:245, 1929. (a)

Wilson, F.: Nursing problems in caring for patients with respiratory disease. *American Journal of Nursing, 29*:520, 1929. (b)

Wilson, F.: Problems in medical care. *American Journal of Nursing, 29*:1049, 1929. (c)

Yura, H., and Walsh, M.: *The Nursing Process: Assessing, Planning, Implementing, Evaluating,* 2nd ed. New York, Appleton-Century Crofts, 1973.

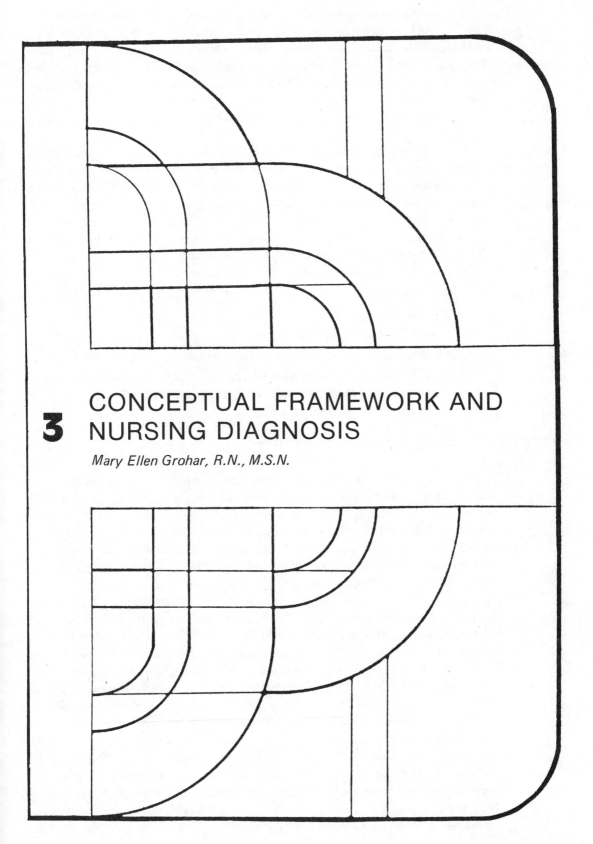

3 CONCEPTUAL FRAMEWORK AND NURSING DIAGNOSIS

Mary Ellen Grohar, R.N., M.S.N.

In its historical and developmental evolution, nursing has advanced to the stage at which its existence and value as an art have been well established. Its reputation as a science is evolving through efforts to define a scientific base of organized knowledge distinct to the nursing profession. These efforts to create a scientific base are reflected most noticeably in the increasing amounts of reported nursing research and articles discussing theory, nursing theory, theoretical frameworks, conceptual frameworks, and conceptual models.

Attempts to gain an understanding of the meaning of these terms through a review of the literature often result in confusion and discouragement because terms are used interchangeably or definitions are vague and inconsistent. While it is not the intent of this chapter to unravel all of the confusion, some of the terminology will be discussed. This chapter will address five questions in the hope that the reader may better understand the relationships between theory, conceptual framework, and nursing process, in particular nursing diagnosis. The questions include:

What is theory?

What is nursing theory?

What is a conceptual framework?

What is the conceptual framework of adaptation used in this text?

What relationships exist between this use of a conceptual framework and nursing process, in particular, nursing diagnosis?

THEORY — ITS MEANING AND IMPORTANCE

In everyday use, the meaning of theory varies from a hunch, or assumption, to an acceptable body of principles offered to explain and predict phenomena (Webster, 1976). The reader is probably better acquainted with the use of the word theory in a casual sense. For example, "theory" is commonly used to describe the content present in classrooms, and while content usually requires some degree of abstraction, it is not appropriately called a theory in the most formal, organized sense.

In a more sophisticated sense, theory is defined as a "system of interrelated propositions used to describe, predict, explain, understand, and control a part of the empirical world" (Roy, 1979). Other experts define theory by classification into types, such as the four levels of theory described by Dickoff and coworkers (1968): factor-isolating theories, factor-relating theories, situation-relating theories, or situation-producing theories. Each of these levels of theories has its own theories, with higher level theory dependent on the theories of lower levels.

Theories are composed of sets of concepts and propositions. Concepts are abstractions, labels attached to objects of study. *Anxiety*, *peace*, *health*, and *illness* are examples of familiar concepts in one's everyday experiences. Propositions are statements of relationship between concepts, relationships that are specific and directional. For example, the statement "continual increases in one's level of *anxiety* directly increase the risk for *illness*" indicates a specific directional relationship between two concepts; therefore it is a proposition. The interrelationship of one or more propositions constitutes the structure of a theory.

The use of theory has its advantages as well as its disadvantages. Theory can represent an entire field of knowledge in essential and concise terms; it becomes a base against which it is possible to test out facts, inaccuracies, and deficiencies; and it can explain as well as predict the phenomenon in question. On the other hand, theory has its disadvantages: theories are developed by men and are, therefore, selective and restrictive in their view. Theories are subject to change as knowledge changes; some theories maintain their usefulness, and others fall into disuse.

NURSING THEORY

The use of theory is not new to nursing; theories from other disciplines have been liberally borrowed by nursing. Systems theory, frequently used in the past, continues to be used as a basis for the construction of nursing models. Similarly, adaptation level theory has been utilized by nurses involved in theory development.

Theories from other disciplines are not always adequate to explain the nature of nursing. This conviction partially accounts for the recent surge of emphasis on theory development for nursing. What is needed are theories of nursing, that is, ways of conceptualizing the nature of nursing as unique, and therefore distinct from other disciplines. Nursing theories are also needed for the service nursing provides, that is, the practice it maintains with clients.

Achievements in the development of nursing theory are occurring more quickly than the literature can report. Some experts believe that the concerted effort by those involved in the nursing diagnostic movement to identify, label, and classify nursing diagnoses is an initial step in theory development (Jacox, 1974). There are increasing numbers of nurse theorists whose works are being tested, refined, and expanded on an ongoing basis. Dorothy Johnson, Dorothea Orem, and Sister Callista Roy are examples of nurse theorists whose works have received widespread attention, discussion, and application. The outcome of these and other theorists' work has promoted the status of nursing theory development, a necessary condition for the advancement of nursing from a discipline to a science.

CONCEPTUAL FRAMEWORK

Other terms frequently occurring in the language of theory are conceptual framework and conceptual model. The terms conceptual framework and conceptual model are usually considered synonymous by most authors. While the use of the word "model" may connote a more visual schema than "framework," this chapter will consider them interchangeably.

A conceptual framework is not a theory in its strictest sense, but provides a way of focusing one's thinking more specifically. A conceptual framework, like a theory, deals with concepts, but in a conceptual framework, the statements of relationships between concepts are not as well defined as in a theory (Polit and Hungler, 1978).

Most of the theoretical work done in nursing has resulted in the development of conceptual frameworks currently being used by nurses (Riehl and Roy, 1980). Such conceptual frameworks are valuable to the development of nursing theory, often serving as the theory's foundation and serving as guides to research, another essential ingredient in theory development. Every conceptual framework is based upon a theory and should include the basic assumptions, values, definitions, and concepts of the theory appropriate to the framework.

Conceptual frameworks used within nursing focus on three elements: the *goal of nursing*, the *client*, and the *manner of nursing action* (Fig. 3–1). Differences in conceptual frameworks reflect not only a difference in theory base but also a difference in interpretation of the meaning of nursing's goal, the client, and nursing action.

Adaptation as a Conceptual Framework*

Adaptation, when used as a conceptual framework, may be defined as the ability of the individual, the family, or the community to modify physiological, psychological, social, cultural, or developmental behaviors to meet health needs. Adaptation is generally viewed as an advantageous change in function of the individual, the family, or the community.

Health corresponds to the situation in which the client (individual, family, or community) responds adaptively. As a dynamic state, health implies the need for continuous adaptation to stimuli through optimum use of resources to achieve maximum potentials. Illness, on the contrary, is an experience during which there is disruption of the adapting mechanisms of the client.

---

*Editor's Note: The conceptual framework of adaptation used in this book has been modified from the model developed and used by the faculty of St. Louis University School of Nursing.

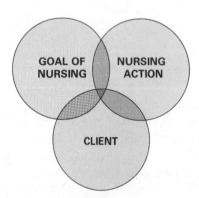

Figure 3–1 Focus of conceptual frameworks.

A determination of the level of adaptation occurs through an assessment of a client's adaptive responses within each of the five adaptive dimensions: physiological, psychological, social, cultural, and developmental. The adaptive response may be adequate, deficient, excessive, inappropriate, or dysfunctional in any or all of the dimensions of behavior. These adaptive responses may have positive or negative consequences in terms of the health of the client. Resources available to the client for adaptation in health and illness are the innate factors of the individual and the support of the family and community.

As is true of any conceptual framework, adaptation has some basic assumptions. They are:

- Adaptation may involve one, several, or all of the dimensions of client behavior.
- Adaptation occurs as a result of a stimulus from the internal or external environment causing a departure from the balanced state.
- Adaptation is an attempt to maintain optimal health conditions within the individual, family, or community.
- The more flexible the individual, family, or community is, the greater the ability to adapt.
- Individuals, families, or communities who use few adaptive mechanisms are limited in their ability to adapt to new and changing situations.

Adaption, as a conceptual framework used in nursing, focuses on three elements: the goal of nursing, the client, and the manner of the nursing action.

The *goal of nursing* is the promotion of the client's adaptation in each of the dimensions of behavior in situations of health and illness. The adaptive responses in each of the dimensions of behavior represent the varying degrees of health or illness. The adaptive level of the client has been determined on the basis of adequate, deficient, excessive, dysfunctional, or inappropriate responses. This adaptive level is the concern of the nurse, and it is her role to facilitate appropriate adaptive resources through the use of the nursing process.

According to the conceptual framework of adaptation, the *client* is the individual, family, or community, who is in constant interaction with the environment (internal or external). To cope with this changing environment the client has innate and acquired resources. The client's responses within the dimensions indicate the level of adaptation. The nurse then analyzes these adaptive responses and plans appropriate nursing care.

In the conceptual framework of adaptation, *nursing action* is the use of the nursing process. The nurse assesses the client in each of the dimensions of behavior and, based on this assessment, determines the adaptive level. Once the adaptive level is determined, the nurse proceeds through the remaining steps of the nursing process.

**Utilization of the Adaptation Framework in the
Nursing Process**

Adaptation is one conceptual framework that can be easily utilized within the nursing process. From information obtained during the *assessment* (history, physical examination, laboratory data) the nurse makes the following determinations within the conceptual framework of adaptation:

1. Identifies alterations in each of the dimensions: physiological, psychological, cultural, developmental, and social.
2. Investigates the client's resources for adapting to change.
3. Judges whether the client's responses are adequate, deficient, excessive, inappropriate, or dysfunctional.

Nursing diagnoses are derived from assessment data within the five adaptive dimensions. The adaptive dimensions provide an efficient means to group data so that information may be interpreted and nursing diagnostic statements formulated. The following examples of nursing diagnoses were formulated according to adaptive dimensions:

Adaptive Dimension	Nursing Diagnosis
Physiological	Fluid volume deficit associated with hemorrhage
Psychological	Anxiety related to hospitalization
Cultural	Impaired communication associated with language barrier
Developmental	Dependency related to chronic illness
Social	Isolation related to lack of transportation

Occasionally, the assessment data from two or more dimensions may be combined to constitute one nursing diagnosis. The following nursing diagnoses were formulated from assessment data from two or more adaptive dimensions:

Adaptive Dimension	Nursing Diagnosis
Psychological and social	Anxiety — moderate, associated with insufficient finances
Developmental and physiological	Impairment of parenting related to acute illness
Physiological, psychological, and cultural	Nutritional alteration related to impaired self-concept subsequent to language barrier.

Nursing diagnostic statements may reflect the adaptive framework by denoting the level of client response to the alteration, using the terms adequate, deficient, excessive, inappropriate, or dysfunctional. When utilizing the conceptual framework of adaptation, the nursing diagnostic label may reflect adaptation terminology but not necessarily.

The *plan* reflects the goal of adaptation — the return of the client to the most positive state of health possible. The plan indicates what will be done to resolve the nursing diagnosis. Knowledge of the client's adaptation state and resources in each dimension enables the plan to be individualized and realistic. For example, the nurse may decide that the plan for one client to lose fifteen pounds in three months may not be realistic for another client who has a similar body structure and height and is just as overweight. Consideration must be given to all five adaptive dimensions and resources available to the client before the plan is developed.

Intervention is the use of specific nursing therapies to assist the client in adaptation. Internal and external resources that are not being utilized to their fullest extent are drafted into action. For example, with a newly diagnosed diabetic, the nurse may assist the client to efficiently utilize his resources by teaching him the relationships between insulin, exercise, and diet. The client's adherence to the instructions hopefully will result in better control of blood sugar and fewer secondary complications from the disease. The external resources of a peer group to discuss ideas, hopes, frustrations, and fears may also be suggested by the nurse to aid in the client's adaptation to illness.

Evaluation within the adaptation framework is the ongoing determination of the client's adaptive status. Determination of the client's adaptive status will dictate whether reassessment or modifications in the nursing diagnosis, plan, and intervention are necessary. For example, the client who was placed on a diet and exercise program with the plan to lose fifteen pounds in three months had lost fifteen pounds but had expressed dissatisfaction with the diet because it restricted a majority of ethnic foods preferred by the client. Thus, evaluation revealed an adequate response within the physiological dimension, but a deficient response in the cultural and social dimensions. Based on this information, the nurse decides that reassessment and formulation of a new nursing diagnosis, plan, intervention, and evaluation is in order.

SUMMARY

This chapter has presented an overview of theory, nursing theory, conceptual framework, and the use of adaptation as a conceptual framework. A realistic utilization of this conceptual framework within the nursing process was also described. It is hoped that an understanding of this information will foster an appreciation of the conceptual work being accomplished in nursing today — work that is essential for the growth of the practice of nursing.

References

Dickoff, J., James, P., and Wiedenbach, E.: Theory in a practice discipline. Part II. Practice oriented research. *Nursing Research*, Nov.–Dec., 1968, p. 545.

Jacox, A.: Theory construction in nursing: An overview. *Nursing Research*, Jan.–Feb., 1974, p. 4.

Polit, D., and Hungler, B.: *Nursing Research: Principles and Methods.* Philadelphia, J.B. Lippincott, 1978.

Riehl, P., and Roy, Sr. C.: *Conceptual Models for Nursing Practice.* New York, Appleton-Century-Crofts, 1980.

Roy, Sr. Callista: *Introduction to Nursing: An Adaptation Model.* Englewood Cliffs, Prentice-Hall, Inc., 1976.

Roy, Sr. Callista: Relating nursing theory to education: A new era. *Nurse Educator*, March–April 1979, p. 16.

St. Louis University School of Nursing. Adaptation Framework, Unpublished, 1980.

Webster's New Collegiate Dictionary. Springfield, Massachusetts, G. & C. Merriam Company, 1976, p. 1209.

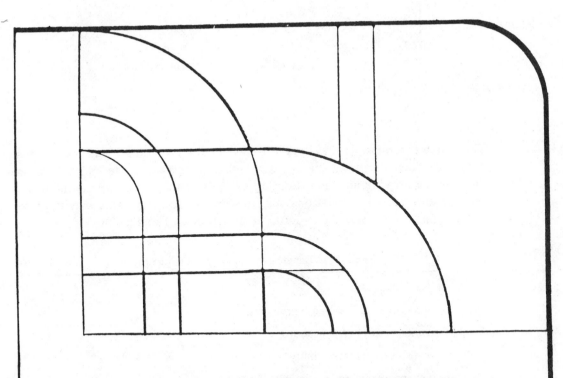

4 ANALYSIS OF THE COMPONENTS OF THE NURSING PROCESS

Anne Griffin Perry, R.N., M.S.N.

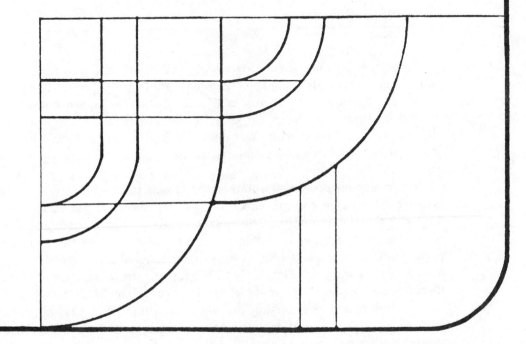

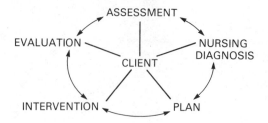

Figure 4-1 Nursing process model.

The nursing process is a systematic method for providing health care. This chapter, which discusses the five-step nursing process model (Fig. 4–1), is designed to provide an understanding of each of the five components of the process and their interrelationships, the knowledge and skills necessary to utilize this process, and the benefits of the process (Table 4–1).

Table 4–1   Benefits of Using the Nursing Process

Creates a health data base.

Identifies actual or potential health problems.

Establishes priorities of nursing action.

Defines specific nursing responsibility.

Develops planned, organized, and individualized nursing care.

Encourages innovative nursing care.

Provides for alternatives of nursing action.

Provides a method for communicating nursing therapies.

Develops nursing autonomy.

Fosters nursing accountability.

Process is defined as a progressive course, moving forward from one point to another while using a detailed methodology (Webster, 1974). Within a process separate components can be identified, but each component is dependent upon and interrelated with the others. Although the nursing process is consistent with Webster's definition of process, it is also characterized by three other important dimensions: *purpose, organization,* and *flexibility.*

The major *purpose* of the nursing process is to provide structure for the delivery of nursing care to meet the health needs of the individual, the family, or the community. The nursing process is *organized* through five sequential components: assessment, diagnosis, plan, intervention, and evaluation. These components provide the organizational structure necessary to accomplish its purpose. *Flexibility* of the nursing process is demonstrated by its applicability to a wide variety of health care recipients.

To understand the nursing process as a whole, it is first necessary to analyze each component as a single unit and then discuss the interrelationships among the components.

ASSESSMENT

The first component of the nursing process, assessment, is a *systematic method of data collection, which consists of the appraisal of the individual, the family, or the community for the purpose of identifying potential and actual health needs*. The data obtained in this phase is collected from a nursing health history, physical examination, and laboratory data. To collect appropriate data during the health history, the nurse must competently utilize the skills of communication and observation. Adequate communication skills enable the nurse to create the comfortable, safe, and therapeutic environment necessary for the assessment phase. To create this type of environment, there must be flexibility as well as an openness in communicating questions to the client in order to elicit appropriate and useful information. While the verbal communication skills are important, the crucial communication skill in conducting the assessment process effectively is listening. Failure of the nurse to listen may result in obtaining incomplete or inaccurate data. In addition, utilization of observation skills is essential to the identification of information in the areas wherein the client does not elaborate fully or declines a response. Observation is essential not only to the health history but to the physical examination as well.

Components of Assessment

Nursing Health History

To obtain a health history the nurse utilizes the client as the primary source of information. However, secondary sources such as family members, significant others, support systems within the community, and other members of the health care team should never be overlooked. These secondary sources can provide the nurse with an abundance of data pertinent to the client's health history, lifestyle, and available adaptive resources within the individual, the family, and the community. While the major objective of the nursing health history is to obtain information about the client's perception of his past and present level of wellness, there are other objectives specific to the nursing health history. Achievement of these objectives provides the nurse with a broad data base pertaining to the client's health status.

Objectives of Nursing Health History

To identify patterns of health and illness

To identify the presence of risk factors for physical and behavioral alterations

To collect data and identify alterations within the adaptive dimensions

To identify available adaptive resources

The health history includes major categories which assist the interviewer in data collection. While there are many ways to obtain a nursing health history, it is important to include the following:

Components of a Nursing Health History

Biographic and demographic information

Client's reason for seeking health care

Client's expectations of health care providers

Client's past and present health status

In eliciting data, an adaptation framework may be used for organizing the information gathered (Fig. 4–2).

In the *physiological dimension* the nurse should utilize sound scientific knowledge to assess the client's physiological responses to alterations in the internal or external environment. In doing this, the nurse identifies the

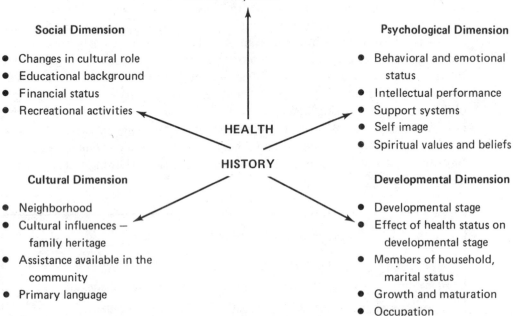

Physiological Dimension

- Past health problems and therapies
- Present health therapies
- Risk factors
- Activity and coordination
- Review of systems

Social Dimension

- Changes in cultural role
- Educational background
- Financial status
- Recreational activities

Psychological Dimension

- Behavioral and emotional status
- Intellectual performance
- Support systems
- Self image
- Spiritual values and beliefs

HEALTH

HISTORY

Cultural Dimension

- Neighborhood
- Cultural influences – family heritage
- Assistance available in the community
- Primary language

Developmental Dimension

- Developmental stage
- Effect of health status on developmental stage
- Members of household, marital status
- Growth and maturation
- Occupation

Figure 4–2 Adaptation framework for gathering a health history.

body's available resources for promoting adaptation, the present stage of physiological adaptation, the inability to adapt to the altered environment, or patterns in the client's family history that may influence adaptation.

It is also important for the nurse to determine psychological adaptation. The nurse assesses how the client copes with actual or potential changes in physiological functioning, changes in family or community structure, and changes in role.

For complete assessment in the *psychological dimension*, the nurse must utilize knowledge of normal and abnormal psychology to evaluate the client's behavioral and emotional status and intellectual performance. Resultant data enables the nurse to identify the client's thought processes, problem-solving abilities, support systems, perception of role and self-image, spiritual needs, and religious practices.

During the health history, the nurse must collect information related to the client's *development*. To do this effectively, the nurse must have knowledge of the behaviors, expectations, needs, and normal role patterns for the various developmental stages of the life cycle. This knowledge provides the nurse with the necessary resources to identify those influences that may hinder or promote appropriate progression through various developmental stages.

Social and *cultural patterns* and their influences should be identified so that the nurse can incorporate them into the nursing care plan. Social and cultural influences can affect (1) the client's willingness to seek out and participate in health care, (2) priorities of health care needs, (3) the type of nursing therapies prescribed, (4) the client's cooperation with therapies, and (5) the client's physiological, psychological, and developmental adaptive responses. The identification of the social and cultural influences challenges the nurse to develop a plan of care that will maximize the client's priorities, values, and social resources. The nurse can further validate this information by data obtained during the physical examination.

Physical Examination

The physical examination is *scrutinization of all body parts through the use of the techniques of inspection, palpation, percussion, and auscultation in search for abnormalities that may yield information concerning present and future health problems.* The major objectives of the physical examination are:

Major Objectives of the Physical Exam

To validate the data obtained in the health history

To identify new assessment data

To differentiate normal from altered findings

To provide a focus for the collection of laboratory data

The examination procedure should be systematic so that all parts of the body are examined, and none are overlooked. The results of the examination, like the details of the history, should be recorded at the time they are elicited so that they are not subject to distortions of memory. Before doing the examination, the nurse should be competent in the techniques of inspection, palpation, percussion, and auscultation and be familiar with normal and abnormal variations. These skills are acquired with time and experience.

Laboratory Data

Another source of assessment information is laboratory data, which provide *supportive validation of alterations identified in the health history and physical examination.* The major objective of laboratory data is to provide baseline information. It is important to incorporate normal as well as altered laboratory findings into the initial assessment data base so that they can be used as standards against which subsequent laboratory results can be compared. Alterations not previously recognized by means of the health history and physical examination may also be identified. The nurse must competently recognize alterations from normal findings and incorporate this data into the client's plan of care.

Use of Assessment Data

While the format for obtaining nursing assessment data may vary from one health-care setting to another and from one nurse to another, the areas of nursing health history, physical examination, and collection of laboratory data should always be considered essential to the assessment process. Upon its completion, the data obtained must be organized so that correct conclusions about the health status of the individual, the family, or the community may be reached. The judgments or conclusions that occur as a result of the collecting and processing of data lead to the formulation of a nursing diagnosis.

A brief clinical example of a client with a respiratory alteration is utilized in Table 4–2 to demonstrate organization of the data obtained in assessment. The data obtained serves as the foundation for the remainder of the nursing process. Mr. Smith is a 50 year old white male admitted to a general medical ward with bilateral lower lobe pneumonia.

NURSING DIAGNOSIS

When all of the health information is compiled, the nurse categorizes pertinent data that reflect alterations in specific areas of adaptation. These alterations, once grouped and labeled, constitute a nursing diagnosis, that is, a *statement of a potential or actual altered health status of a client(s), which is derived from nursing assessment and which requires intervention from the domain of nursing practice.* Each nursing diagnosis should be stated

Table 4–2 Pertinent Assessment Data from Mr. Smith

Physiological	Psychological	Cultural	Developmental	Social
		Health History		
This is the first hospitalization, with no history of health problems. Last physical examination was 3 months ago. Father died at age 65 of stomach cancer; one brother died at age 40 of heart attack. Rest of family history is negative. Does not smoke or drink alcohol or coffee. Plays tennis 3 times week.	Wife described their 25 years of marriage as close, no major problems. Mr. Smith stated that being ill made him "angry" because he was unable to do his normal activities. He and his wife are very active in social, business, and religious activities of the Baptist church.	Lives with wife in a suburban neighborhood. The Smiths and the majority of their neighbors have lived there for 15 years. He describes the neighborhood as upper middle class and professional people.	A chemist at a major drug firm for the last 25 years. Complete hospitalization coverage. Appears to be a mature adult, accepting responsibilities and anticipating no changes because of illness.	Doctorate in chemistry. No financial difficulties. He and his wife travel every 1-2 months on business. They camp every summer with their daughters and families.
		Physical Examination		
Cardiac: Rate 114/minute. B.P. 110/80. Temp: 102°F orally. No abnormal sounds or rubs. Pulses equal. Respiratory: Rate 38/min. Decreased breath sounds and decreased excursion bilaterally. Sputum: green, foul odor.	Facial expressions and gestures appropriate.		Height: 6' 4" Weight: 220 lbs. Muscle mass: well developed. No evidence of any skeletal or structural abnormalities. Verbal responses appropriate for adult developmental stage.	
		Laboratory Data		
Chest x-ray: Bilateral lower lobe consolidation. Sputum: multiple *Diplococcus pneumoniae* organisms. Hemoglobin: 11 mg/100 ml Hematocrit: 33%				

accurately, based on current conclusions derived from the health history, physical examination, and laboratory studies.

The incorporation of the nursing diagnosis within the nursing process provides a central focus for the nursing plans; interventions, and evaluations. In addition, the nursing diagnosis offers an efficient form of communication and specific directions for nursing interventions. It is also invaluable in promoting consistency of nursing care, identifying the domain of nursing practice, and providing effective avenues for establishing accountability.

In order to arrive at an accurate nursing diagnosis, the nurse must have completed an accurate and complete health assessment that can be patterned into diagnostic categories. This requires that the nurse have a strong scientific knowledge base and an understanding of a conceptual framework of nursing. An illustration of how nursing diagnosis flows from the assessment data is portrayed in Table 4-3.

Table 4-3 Client Example of Nursing Diagnoses Derived from Assessment Data

	Assessment Data	Nursing Diagnoses
Health History	"Cold for one month." First hospitalization. Productive cough for one week. Sputum "green, odorous." Fever for 10 days; range: 100.8 to 102°F orally, not relieved with aspirin.	Altered ventilation related to retained secretions. Alterations in role related to illness and hospitalization. Increased nutritional requirements related to prolonged fever.
Physical Examination	Decreased breath sounds in left and right lower lobes. Decreased respiratory excursion. Moist rales (crackles) bilaterally. Productive cough. Tenacious, green, odorous sputum. Respiratory rate: 32/min.	Potential alterations in oxygenation related to decreased lung expansion and decreased hemoglobin.
Laboratory Data	Chest x-ray shows bilateral consolidation in lower lobes. Sputum culture shows *Diplococcus pneumoniae.* Hemoglobin: 11mg/100 ml Hematocrit: 33%	

PLAN

The plan consists of the *determination by the nurse and client of those goals that must be achieved to promote adaptation.* Planning involves goal-setting and establishing priorities.

In assisting with goal formulation the client needs to identify those goals that are important to him in facilitating adaptation. The goals need to be individualized for each client and he or she must help determine priorities. While the goal-setting and priority selection indicate what will be done, nursing intervention provides the methodology for accomplishing the goal.

An illustration of the plan for Mr. Smith's first nursing diagnosis, *altered ventilation related to retained secretions,* is presented in Table 4-4.

Table 4-4 Client Example of Plan Developed from Nursing Diagnosis

	Assessment Data	Nursing Diagnosis	Plan
Health History	"Cold for one month." Productive cough for one week. Sputum "green, odorous."		
Physical Examination	Decreased breath sounds in left and right lower lobes. Moist rales (crackles) bilaterally. Productive cough. Tenacious, green, odorous sputum. Respiratory rate 32/min.	Altered ventilation related to retained secretions.	**To elimate retained respiratory secretions.**
Laboratory Data	Chest x-ray shows bilateral consolidation in lower lobes. Sputum culture shows *Diplococcus pneumoniae.*		

INTERVENTION

Intervention is the *use of nursing therapies necessary to accomplish the defined plans and to promote adaptation of the individual, the family, and the community.* Prior to the actual implementation of interventions, the nurse must be competent in three general areas: (1) knowledge, which provides the scientific rationale for selected nursing interventions; (2) knowledge of the health care system so that the nurse can identify additional health care resources to assist the client in achieving adaptation; and (3) psychomotor skills that the nurse can utilize in implementing the planned interventions.

Table 4-5 incorporates the specific nursing interventions selected to promote adaptation for Mr. Smith in relation to the plan established.

Table 4–5 Client Example of Nursing Interventions Used to Achieve Plan

	Assessment Data	Nursing Diagnosis	Plan	Intervention
Health History	"Cold for one month." Productive cough for one week. Sputum "green, odorous."			
Physical Examination	Decreased breath sounds in left and right lower lobes. Moist rales (crackles) bilaterally. Productive cough. Tenacious, green, odorous sputum. Respiratory rate 32/min.	Altered ventilation related to retained secretions.	To eliminate retained respiratory secretions.	Elevate the head of the bed 45°. Turn, deep breathe, and cough every 2 hours. Postural drainage twice a day. Rest periods scheduled. Increase fluid intake to 2000cc each 24 hours.
Laboratory Data	Chest x-ray shows bilateral consolidation in lower lobes. Sputum culture shows *Diplococcus pneumoniae.*			

EVALUATION

Evaluation, the last component of the nursing process, is the *ongoing measurement of goal achievement in relation to the stated nursing diagnoses.* Evaluation involves three activities: (1) the statement of criteria by which goal achievement is determined, frequently called outcome criteria; (2) the gathering of a data base about which a statement of goal achievement can be made; and (3) the actual statement of judgment about degree of goal achievement.

If evaluation discloses unmet goals, the nurse must review the entire nursing process step-by-step to verify the accuracy of each step. Such continued investigation may reveal errors or omissions in assessment, diagnosis, plan, or intervention. Once appropriate corrective measures are instituted, the sequence of nursing process activities continues.

The competencies required of the professional nurse in evaluating a care plan include the ability to develop evaluative criteria, to gather a data base upon which a goal achievement statement can be made, and to form and articulate judgments. Further, if goal achievement is not accomplished, the nurse must utilize the skills of assessment to investigate the reasons and modify the previous approach to the client.

It is difficult to represent the entire process of evaluation in the traditional nursing care plan. Often what is represented is the list of evaluative or outcome criteria, but other approaches include the actual statement of judgment or a description of the data base upon which judgment is made.

Table 4–6 represents the incorporation of the evaluation component into the care plan for Mr. Smith in the form of outcome criteria.

INTERRELATIONSHIPS AMONG THE COMPONENTS OF THE NURSING PROCESS

Up to this point, the components of the nursing process have been studied as singular units. However, for understanding of the process and its application to health care settings, interrelationships among components must be discussed. Process suggests action and systematic movement in order to arrive at a desired goal. Also inherent in the definition of process is the concept of a unified whole that, in the case of nursing, can be described in terms of components, with each component related to the other (Figure 4–3). By itself, each component is an artificial separation of actions; in nursing practice such separation cannot realistically be achieved. An understanding of the interrelatedness of the components of the nursing process gives the nurse the opportunity to create change, individualize nursing care, strengthen nursing knowledge, allow for flexibility, and practice in a variety of health care settings.

The components of the nursing process follow a logical progression, with each component dependent on the other. During the **assessment** phase, the nurse gathers data that designate differing levels of adaptation, and this

Table 4–6 Client Example of Evaluation

	Assessment Data	Nursing Diagnosis	Plan	Intervention	Evaluation
Health History	"Cold for one month." Productive cough for one week. Sputum "green, odorous."	Altered ventilation related to retained secretions.	To eliminate retained respiratory secretions.	Elevate the head of the bed 45°. Turn, deep breathe, and cough every 2 hours. Postural drainage to all lobes twice a day. Periods of rest. Increase fluid intake to 2000cc each 24 hours.	Increased breath sounds while head of bed elevated. Decreased rales (crackles) after turning, coughing, and deep breathing and postural drainage. Absence of rales (crackles) after three postural drainage treatments. Decrease in sputum production; sputum clearing.
Physical Examination	Decreased breath sounds in left and right lower lobes. Moist rales (crackles) bilaterally. Productive cough. Tenacious, green odorous sputum. Respiratory rate 32/min.				
Laboratory Data	Chest x-ray shows bilateral consolidation in lower lobes. Sputum culture shows *Diplococcus pneumoniae.*				Normal temperature. Clearing chest x-ray. Adequate 24-hour fluid intake and output.

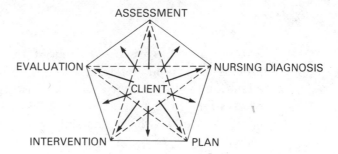

Figure 4-3 Interrelationship of components of nursing process.

culminates in the formulation of the nursing diagnosis. The nursing diagnosis is not possible without assessment data. The assessment phase gives the nurse the opportunity to gather data that identify and label the client's degree of wellness or illness. Without this data there is insufficient information for the nurse to form a conclusion about the health status of the client. Following the grouping of data and the formulation of a nursing diagnosis, the data provide the basis for developing a plan of care based on *priorities* and possible successes of each plan. During intervention, the focus is on the *methodology* and nursing actions needed to maintain or change the adaptational level of the client. Evaluation is used to *verify* the client's expected response to planned actions. The elements of evaluation are concurrent and recurrent based on the goal achievement. Assessment, therefore, must articulate with each of the components of the nursing process.

Nursing diagnosis is an organized *concluding* statement derived from assessment data, which infers the setting of priorities during the planning phase of the nursing process. The nursing diagnosis indicates whether and what type of nursing *actions* will be taken to alter the adaptation level of the client. The evaluation statement verifies the accuracy and effectiveness of the nursing diagnosis.

The **planning** phase of the process allows the nurse to *designate* specific actions to be taken by the nurse and provides the framework for the *outcomes* during evaluation of the health care given. The plan could not be developed without *interpretation* of the assessment data and the *establishment* of a nursing diagnosis.

Via the *avenue* of assessment and depending on the stated nursing diagnosis, the *organization* of priorities, and the planned *methodology*, **nursing intervention** take place. Evaluation indicates the *accuracy* of the outcomes of nursing interventions.

Evaluation allows for *validation* of the expected outcomes and gives *direction* and *indicators* for reassessing, establishing *accuracy* of nursing diagnoses, reorganizing priorities, and selecting alternate nursing action in order to meet the client's nursing care needs.

SUMMARY

This chapter has discussed each of the five components of the nursing process and their interrelationships. An example of a client with an alteration in respiratory status was incorporated to demonstrate the progression through the nursing process from assessment to evaluation. In addition, the knowledge and skills necessary to utilize the process have been presented.

References

Aspinall, M.J.: Nursing diagnosis — the weak link. *Nursing Outlook, 24:*433. 1976.

Banathy, B.J.: *Instructional Systems.* Palo Alto, California: Fearon, 1968.

Bevis, E.O.: *Curriculum Building in Nursing a Process.* St. Louis: C.V. Mosby Co., 1978.

Bircher, A.U.: On the development and classification of diagnoses. *Nursing Forum,* 14:11, 1975.

Carrieri, V.K., and Sitzman, J.: Components of the nursing process. *Nursing Clinics of North America, 6:*115, 1971.

Gordon, M.: Classification of nursing diagnoses. *Journal New York State Nurses Association, 9:*5, 1978.

Gordon, M.: Nursing diagnosis and the diagnostic process. *American Journal of Nursing,* 76:1298, 1976.

Hefferin, E., and Hunter, R.E.: Nursing assessment and care plan statements. *Nursing Research 24:*360, 1975.

Judge, R., and Zuidema, G. *Physical Diagnosis: A Physiologic Approach to the Clinical Examination,* 2nd ed. Boston: Little, Brown and Co., 1963.

Maas, M., Spechet, J., and Jacox, A.: Nurse autonomy reality not rhetoric. *American Journal of Nursing, 75:*2201, 1975.

Von Bertalanffy, L.: *General Systems Theory Foundations, Development and Application.* New York: George Braziller, Inc., 1968.

Webster's New School and Office Dictionary. Greenwich, Connecticut: Fawcett Publications, Inc., 1975.

Yura, H., and Walsh, M.B.: *The Nursing Process,* 3rd ed. New York: Appleton-Century-Crofts, 1978.

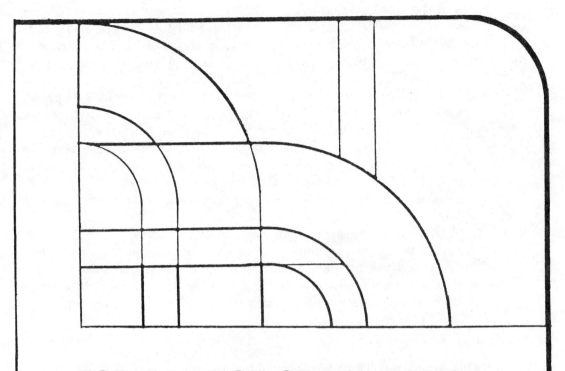

5 FORMULATION OF A NURSING DIAGNOSIS

Marion M. Resler, R.N., M.S.N.

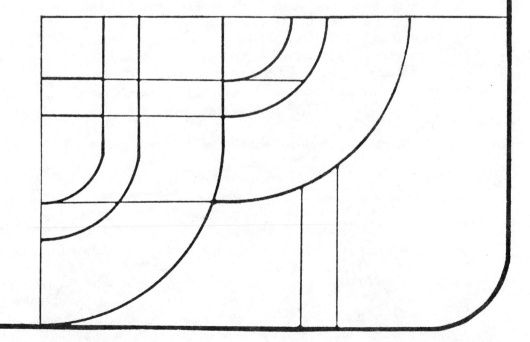

Previous chapters explored the importance of nursing diagnosis as a distinct step in the nursing process. This chapter will focus on the nursing diagnosis itself — how it is formulated and stated and how nursing knowledge is applied to each event in the diagnostic sequence to ensure accuracy, appropriateness, and usefulness.

At first thought, the method of diagnosis may seem obvious — a matter of categorizing the assessment and making a statement about it. In practice, however, there is much confusion among nurses about this "categorizing and stating" process. The most important requirement of a statement of nursing diagnosis is that it be based on consideration of all pertinent, available information, so that it will lead logically to an appropriate plan, intervention, and evaluation. A nursing diagnosis based on incomplete information may be useless or misleading and may cause errors or omissions in the plan of care.

Formulating a nursing diagnosis is a problem-solving process not unlike the problem solving that nurses use in much of their work. It is guided by the judicious use of nursing knowledge every step of the way from the nursing assessment, which is the first step, to the statement of diagnosis, which is the product of the analysis and interpretation of the information gathered in assessment.

THE DEVELOPMENT OF NURSING KNOWLEDGE

Many nurses — students and practitioners alike — express feelings of being unable to formulate a nursing diagnosis. They often cite lack of experience or lack of advanced education as the basis for their difficulty. In reality, all professional nurses possess or have access to much *nursing knowledge* that will help them to gather data and to organize and interpret it in a way that will lead to accurate and useful nursing diagnoses.

Webster's Third New International Dictionary of the English Language, Unabridged (1971) defines knowledge, in part, as "acquaintance with or theoretical or practical understanding of some branch of science, art, learning, or other area involving study, research, or practice and the acquisition of skills." All of these components and characteristics are found in nursing knowledge.

Nursing knowledge has evolved and accumulated over many years and contains facts and information from many disciplines. Nursing is heavily influenced by what is known about the anatomical and biochemical structure of man as well as by knowledge of physiological, psychological, social, cultural, and developmental function. Study of the humanities has also contributed another dimension to nursing knowledge. The depth of understanding of human beings has grown with knowledge of the historical perspective surrounding our existence. Literature also has enriched the understanding of man's response to infirmity and to grief and has described man's hopes and joys and frustrations. In recent times, nurses have turned more frequently to the philosopher and theologian as they struggle with the ethical dilemmas presented by the tremendous advances in science.

All of these disciplines have contributed knowledge to the practice of nursing. Nurses have questioned, researched, and validated their practice over time and have added to the unique body of knowledge. Because nursing knowledge has evolved and developed in this way, the student or practicing nurse is able to approach the task of nursing diagnosis with knowledge previously learned through study and experience, plus nursing knowledge available from a wide variety of other sources.

Use of Knowledge in Assessment and Nursing Diagnosis

Use of knowledge begins with the first interaction between nurse and client. During the initial introductions and explanations an "on-the-spot" assessment is done as the nurse observes the client. This interaction may require use of knowledge to meet the needs of the client even before the formal data collection is initiated. As more structured data gathering is carried out and diagnoses are formulated, nursing knowledge continues to be used in several ways.

Identification of Priorities

Example: A nursing student, Ms. Jones, has been assigned to a newly admitted hospital patient. During the assessment she notes that the patient responds to her conversation with short, gasping phrases. Using her knowledge of physiological alterations that might affect respiration, she assesses for pain or injury; examines skin color, temperature, and moisture of face and extremities; auscultates breath sounds and blood pressure; measures the rate and observes the quality of pulse and respirations; and obtains a short history and description of this alteration from the patient. This ability to identify priorities enables her to initiate appropriate interventions quickly. When the patient's distress has been relieved, she will be able to proceed with the gathering of other data.

Determination of Areas That Need Greater Assessment

Example: While interviewing a new client at the neighborhood health center, the nurse, Mr. Smith, learns that the client has a twenty-year history of poorly controlled diabetes mellitus. Using his knowledge of vascular alterations associated with diabetes, the nurse makes sure that the examination includes careful inspection of legs, feet, and shoes, assessment of the client's knowledge of foot care, and a thorough ophthalmic examination. He will also include an in-depth evaluation of oxygenation and nutrition status.

Interpretation of Data.

Example: Ms. Price, a community health nurse, notes that one of the clients she is visiting takes both a digitalis preparation and a potent diuretic daily. Knowing that potassium depletion may occur with some diuretic therapy, and that this may increase the risk of digitalis toxicity, she consults a pharmacology reference to determine whether the diuretic preparation her patient is receiving could have this effect. Finding that it could, she refreshes her knowledge about digitalis toxicity and uses the knowledge to decide whether the findings of her assessment include data suggestive of digitalis toxicity.

These examples illustrate that use of knowledge facilitates accurate assessment and diagnosis in two ways. First, it guides the direction of the assessment by identifying areas of priority. Second, it enables the nurse to interpret significant data for the purpose of diagnosis. The nurse will use knowledge that has been acquired from study and experience as well as knowledge that is available in the nursing literature and from resource persons. When approaching the task of nursing diagnosis, the nurse applies this knowledge in a problem-solving way, recognizes when additional knowledge is needed, and knows where it may be found.

DATA COLLECTION

A critical ingredient of the formulation of accurate and useful nursing diagnoses is the effective and appropriate collection of *assessment data!* Error in diagnosis is most often the result of errors or omissions in the data collection. This results in nursing diagnoses based on only the most obvious or incomplete data.

Example: A 68 year old man was admitted to the hospital with a medical diagnosis of poorly controlled diabetes mellitus. It was felt by the nursing staff that more education was needed. They noted that the man agreed readily to everything that was said but appeared to lose interest quickly. The staff felt that he did not take his condition seriously. A nursing diagnosis was made on the basis of this behavior: *nonadherence to the diabetes regimen related to lack of motivation.*

Teaching was directed toward stressing the importance and seriousness of careful maintenance of the regimen with detailed explanations of the complications that might result if he failed to do so. Contrary to expectation, the patient's behavior did not change as the teaching progressed.

A nursing student caring for him reviewed the current and previous hospital charts and noted that this man had a long history of various types of vascular disorders. She spoke with the patient's wife and learned that he had been demonstrating increased memory loss and some changes in behavior. The nursing student next consulted the physician, who indicated that he felt the patient's altered intellectual function was related to vascular disease. When the student added this information to the nursing assessment data, it resulted in a revised and more appropriate diagnosis: *reduced ability to carry out the diabetes regimen related to altered cerebral function.*

The nursing student consulted the literature for information about effective health teaching of persons with impairment of cerebral function. The teaching plan was revised; shorter, more simplified sessions were provided and simple visual aids were prepared. The patient's wife was included in the teaching sessions. The revised nursing diagnosis and plan resulted in an improvement in the patient's ability to carry out parts of the regimen such as urine testing, and provision was made for help with the more complex tasks such as insulin administration and diet planning.

Requirements for Effective Collection of Assessment Data

The nurse will proceed with data collection in a manner that will provide information to enable the formulation of accurate, useful nursing diagnoses. To accomplish this purpose, the data collection must be systematic, as comprehensive as possible, and appropriate to the situation.

The nurse meets these requirements by employing the following practices during the data collection process:

1. Utilization of all possible sources of data
2. Use of an assessment tool or outline
3. Use of effective methodology
4. Adjustment of all aspects of the process to the needs of the client, the situation, and the setting

Sources of Assessment Data

Sources of assessment data vary with the client, the situation, and the setting. The following are usual sources of data:

- Interview
- Observation
- Physical Examination
- Laboratory Data
- Records
- Consultation

Interview

The nurse should interview the client as early as possible in the assessment process and explain to the client in simple terms the purpose of the nursing assessment and what it will include. Clients should understand that they are participants in the planning of nursing care that is tailored to their needs and priorities and that, in order to do this, they must supply information and express concerns about their health care. To make the interview meaningful, the nurse must utilize effective interview skills, including the ability to adapt the interview technique to each situation. There are many resources available to the nurse that describe in-depth interview techniques utilizing principles of effective communication. Sometimes, it is also necessary or desirable, within legal and ethical boundaries, to interview a member or members of the client's family or a friend or neighbor to obtain data that the client is unable to supply and to gain additional insights into the health need and its effect on the client and others.

Observation

Some observations that the nurse makes during assessment include the general appearance, facial expression, and grooming of the client; posture, gait, and body language; and behaviors and mannerisms. The nurse should be sensitive to the subtleties of verbal and non-verbal communication. She should note the client's behavior during interaction with staff and with friends and family as well as changes in behavior in response to pain and stress or to changes in the situation or environment. There are more specific observations that the nurse will make as assessment progresses. Some of these observations are made as part of the physical examination.

Physical Examination

The nurse's qualifications to do a physical examination vary with her background, education, and experience. Even the beginning nursing student is able to do parts of the examination such as assessment of vital signs; measurement of height, body weight, and circumference of extremities; and visual inspection of the skin and musculoskeletal system. The nurse in the expanded role may do the entire physical examination and share findings with the physician responsible for the medical aspect of the client's health care. In any setting, the nurse should ensure that provision is made for the physical examination and should share with other members of the health team information from the assessment that would suggest areas in which further or more sophisticated examination might be required. Care should be taken to avoid overlooking data from physical examinations performed by other members of the health team.

The complete physical examination to determine general health status may be done in a head to toe order or in a system by system format. The physical examination may be focused in depth upon an area where there is an alteration present — for example, a person experiencing pain in the abdomen would be examined thoroughly in relation to that symptom, while the rest of the complete examination might be deferred until the immediate need was met.

Laboratory Data

Included in the nurse's assessment will be relevant data from laboratory tests and other diagnostic studies that the client may have undergone. Laboratory studies may range from routine analysis of blood and urine to specialized studies such as pulmonary function tests, x-ray examinations, tissue biopsies, electrocardiography, electroencephalography, and psychological tests. The nurse will use knowledge to interpret and evaluate the *significance* of laboratory data in terms of the adaptive status of the client.

Records

The client in any health care setting will have a written record in which biographical data, information about health status, and a record of health interventions are documented. When caring for clients, the nurse should be thoroughly knowledgeable about the information on the record and should be conscientious about reviewing it regularly. Past records of hospitalizations and other health care interventions should always be reviewed because they can provide valuable insights into the person's *long-term* health status.

The format and subject matter of records found in various health care agencies will depend upon the organization and purpose of each agency. Whatever the setting, the nursing assessment is incomplete without the information that is found in the client's health care records. With experience, the nurse becomes able to review health records for significant data quickly and efficiently.

Consultation

Consultation carried out by the nurse during the process of assessment and diagnosis includes not only persons and literature related to nursing, but also persons and literature related to other disciplines. The nurse consults personally with other members of the health team such as the physician, social worker, nutritionist, pharmacist, physical therapist, and chaplain. She also finds that the literature of these professionals is a valuable source of information, as are textbooks and periodicals related to the physical and social sciences. In addition, there are many community educational and service resources that supply technical information about a particular health-related problem.

The Assessment Form

There are many types of nursing assessment forms, outlines, or tools available. Some of them are very lengthy and complete; others merely designate major categories of function and living with which nurses are concerned. Most health care institutions and agencies have an assessment form unique to their needs. Nursing students may be given a form that is used by their school, or in some cases, they may be expected to design their own assessment form.

Whether the assessment form is long and detailed or short and concise is a matter of individual preference. What *is* most essential is that provision is made to gather data about *all* aspects of the client's health status and health history, as well as relevant data about family, home, and community. It is important to remember that nursing assessment is not a one-time thing — to be useful and safe, the assessment must be ongoing and current. This makes it necessary to provide space for additional entries as new data becomes available. Clients should always have the opportunity to contribute anything they consider significant about their health status and their lives. They should be encouraged to verbalize their understanding of their health needs and their expectations of outcome for the health care that is to be given.

Effective Methodology for Data Collection

The inexperienced nurse may assume that it is desirable to begin data collection by starting at the first line of the assessment form and proceeding with great determination through every line until the end has been reached.

This may result in having some sort of notation in each space, but will not assure effective assessment. In many situations the nurse may wish to begin the data collection by reviewing the client's current health records and recording significant data onto the assessment form. This will not only provide some information before beginning the interview, but will prevent asking the client questions that have already been answered. It will also enable the nurse to clarify or validate information from the records with the help of the client. The nurse may also seek information from other health care workers who have knowledge of the client that would facilitate the interview.

The patient interview should begin with what the client perceives to be most important. This usually involves the health concern responsible for the client being in the health care setting. *If the client's priority health concerns are not addressed promptly, he or she will have little patience with the data collection process and will not understand its value.*

Example: An energetic 73 year old woman who lived alone was admitted to the hospital because she had fallen in her home several times during the previous week. This was of tremendous concern to her because she valued her independence and wished to continue to live in her own home. Before the interview, the nursing student reviewed the chart and noted on the assessment form that the patient's blood sugar levels were at the lowest limits of the normal range. She began the interview by focusing on the client's reason for seeking health care, the falls, and learned that they had been preceded by dizziness.

This led to an exploration of other health problems experienced by the client. She mentioned taking "a pill for diabetes" each morning, although no such pill was being given in the hospital. A nutrition history and information about the client's lifestyle revealed that she often omitted meals. At this point, the nursing student discussed with the patient plans to consult the physician about the oral hypoglycemics taken at home and to work with the nutritionist to develop a practical food plan. Talking with the client about management of her diabetes led easily to the other areas of assessment such as skin integrity, circulatory status, and sensory function.

Data gathered during the assessment will be of two types: subjective and objective. Subjective data (symptoms) will be what the client says or describes or perceives, for example, a statement about pain. This type of statement should be recorded in a way that identifies it clearly as subjective data. For example, *client states, "I have this terrible pain in my side that travels to my back,"* or *client describes pain in right side radiating to the right flank.* It should *not* be recorded *client has pain in the right side.* Objective data (signs) are what the nurse or others observe, measure, or determine, and are stated as specifically and concisely as possible. For example, *client is moaning and massaging left flank; face is pale, cold, and moist; radial pulse 110, regular, thready; blood pressure 140/85.*

Nurses are often more comfortable collecting data about physiological alterations than they are seeking information about the psychological, cultural, developmental, and social status of the client. Nursing diagnoses will be inaccurate if these dimensions are not included. Collecting this kind of data will be less stressful if the nurse does not ask personal questions at the beginning of the interview. Many assessment forms place these categories first, but it is not usually necessary or desirable to initiate the interview this way. If questions of a personal nature are postponed until the rest of the interview has been completed, the nurse will know what kinds of personal data are really needed and will be able to explain to the client how this information will be used. Much of the information may already have been provided during the course of the interview.

When it is necessary to know personal information very quickly to plan needed interventions, assuring the client that this information will be used objectively and discretely can do much to facilitate the sharing of sensitive information. Examples of this type of information that might be needed immediately include instances when the presence of alcohol or street drugs in the bloodstream would increase risks associated with medical or nursing therapies (for example, administration of anesthetics or narcotic analgesics) or when the possibility of pregnancy must be considered before planning diagnostic tests that would expose the client to radiation.

An area of assessment that is sometimes overlooked is the client's developmental status. Each developmental stage includes tasks to be completed. Changes in the client's health status may prohibit completion of current developmental tasks or may require performance of tasks usually addressed in a later developmental stage.

Example: A 70 year old woman was scheduled for emergency surgery for a life-threatening aortic aneurysm. A developmental task for her involved maintaining contact with loved ones. However, the nurse learned through the assessment that the woman had become alienated from family and friends. She now faced serious surgery without any support system. A part of the nurse's care plan for this woman included designing a support system utilizing neighborhood, church, and community resources.

Example: A 50 year old man's deteriorating health status forced him into the *next* developmental stage. Though he had not yet successfully completed the tasks of middle age, he had to face additional tasks that are normally a part of old age. One of these tasks involved finding a more sheltered place to live out his remaining years. Having identified this developmental conflict, the nurse was better able to interpret the client's behavior, make a diagnosis, plan intervention, and evaluate the care plan.

Adjusting the Data Collection Process to the Situation

Major factors to be considered when evaluating the situation in which a nursing assessment is to be done are the *urgency* of the situation, the *environment or care setting,* the *purpose* for which the client is seeking health care, and the *uniqueness of the client* himself.

Types of information that will help the nurse to determine the urgency of the situation include physical signs the client may be demonstrating, medical diagnoses, and laboratory data. When the client is in pain or respiratory distress, the assessment must be quickly and efficiently directed toward areas of priority, with a minimal expenditure of energy from the client. Other sources of data must be used as much as possible. This is also true when a medical diagnosis or laboratory findings indicate that alterations exist which would make a lengthy assessment stressful to the client's adaptation status.

The health care setting and purposes for which the client is seeking care also determine the method and format of data collection. Assessment is always directed toward the client as a total person, but each setting has additional areas of priority. The following is a very brief overview of assessment in some specific settings.

The assessment of the person admitted to the *emergency room or critical care unit* is a "first things first" situation. Evaluation of patency of the airway is first and foremost, followed by determination of effectiveness of respiration and circulation. Then, other life-threatening alterations are investigated and interventions initiated as quickly as possible to maintain function of vital organs and systems. The total assessment may not be completed for days because of the urgent nature of some alterations.

For the patient who enters the hospital with an acute condition, the assessment will be directed first to the purpose for which the person has entered the hospital. With the *routine medical admission*, the nurse will make the assessment as broad as possible and will spend extra time on priority areas. The patient entering the hospital for *scheduled surgery* will be assessed for general physical and mental health status and specifically for his understanding of the surgery to be done, as well as his learning readiness for pre-operative and post-operative teaching. His support system should be described so that post-operative care and rehabilitation can be planned. Alterations and factors that would increase risks associated with surgery and anesthesia should be identified.

The assessment of the client in the *community setting* is directed initially toward the area of greatest concern, but also toward family and community strengths and weaknesses. The maintenance of optimal health and the prevention of illness is a major focus of nursing in the community setting, so the nurse must identify the client's and family's usual means for obtaining health care and their methods of coping with stress. The nurse also looks for economic, social, and environmental factors that may affect the health status and health behavior of the client and family.

There will be occasions in any setting when early completion of the assessment will not be possible because of *constraints on the nurse's time.* In this case, as in emergency situations, the nurse must immediately direct assessment to major alterations and priorities and to the client's chief concerns.

Characteristics and behaviors of the client may require adjustment of the data collection process. There are times when the client communicates verbally or non-verbally that he wishes to be left alone. The nurse should verbalize recognition of this communication and should modify the interview appropriately. When the interview with the client has to be short for *any* reason, the nurse has to be resourceful with powers of observation, examination skills, and the use of records, resource persons, and the literature.

Occasionally, *altered intellectual function, decreased level of consciousness, a communication disorder, or a language barrier* may prevent the client from supplying information about his health status. It is possible to do an effective nursing assessment under even these circumstances. When the client has an altered level of consciousness or mental function, it may be necessary to arrange an interview with a family member, a friend, or a neighbor to obtain whatever health history or other data they can supply. All charts and records, new and old, must be searched for data, and information should be sought from other health care workers who have knowledge of the person.

When there is a communication disorder such as aphasia, it is necessary for the nurse to understand the nature of the disorder in order to work out a system of communication. The speech therapist can be a valuable resource in this situation. When there is a language barrier, it is frequently possible to find someone who will serve as interpreter. If not, simple terms can be identified for client and nurse to use together. It is true in almost any situation and setting that the nurse who demonstrates a sincere desire to communicate effectively with the client will find that the client responds by communicating as effectively as he or she can.

Use of Assessment Data to Identify Alterations of Adaptation

The nurse, having completed all the steps of data collection, will proceed with the integration and interpretation of the collected data in order to identify alterations or potential alterations of adaptation. These alterations form the bases for nursing diagnoses.

A nursing diagnosis is usually a two-part statement. The first part deals with the *alteration* of adaptation related to health status experienced by the client. The second part is concerned with the *reason* for the alteration and gives direction to nursing action. Diagnoses written by nurses deal most often with the *responses to* or *effects of* the alteration in health status. For example, a person who has sustained an injury may be experiencing effects and responses such as pain, reduced mobility, change in ability to carry out the activities of daily living, interruption of income, and change in family role. These responses and effects alter the adaptive status of the person and thus form the bases for nursing diagnoses. The structure of the diagnostic statement will be described later in this chapter. This section discusses the process used to identify alterations of adaptation for which the nurse will write nursing diagnoses.

Many nurses consider the interpretation and integration of data to be the most troublesome part of the diagnostic process because it requires much analytical thinking as well as transfer of theoretical knowledge to situations that often seem unclear. The key to successful interpretation and integration of assessment data is the *careful review* of the assessment data. If gaps are found when the data are reviewed, they should be filled if possible. If some of the data seem contradictory, illogical, or difficult to understand, the nurse should take time to further assess the client, consult with another member of the health team, or make use of a reference source.

As the assessment data is reviewed, it must be judged against knowledge of the structure, function, and adaptive dimensions of the individual — physiological, psychological, cultural, developmental, and social. Findings will be noted that are suggestive of *adaptive responses that are not adequate or are excessive, deficient, or dysfunctional.*

To facilitate the assessment process, the nurse may find it helpful to make a list of every assessment finding that seems to be significant. Medical diagnoses, if any, should be on the list, as well as comments about the client's own perception of his health status and adaptive capacity. Such a list may reveal that there are relationships or trends among the data, and that some of the data form a pattern. Sometimes, the relationship will be within one adaptive dimension, but more often findings from several adaptive dimensions are related.

For example, the presence of dyspnea, pallor or cyanosis, and decreased energy reserve will suggest a pattern related to alteration in oxygenation. All of these assessment findings occur within the physiological dimension that includes circulation, ventilation, and respiration. In another situation, the nurse may discover that a change in a client's digestion and elimination functions began with the longer working hours and irregular eating patterns associated with a new, more demanding job. Here, data from the physiological dimension combine with data from the psychological and social dimensions to form a pattern.

When a relationship appears to exist among several findings of assessment, as in the examples just given, the nurse will wish to establish the significance of the relationship for the purpose of diagnosis. This may be done by clarifying or adding to the data gathered, by consultation, or by use of the literature.

Example: Miss N., a nurse in a neighborhood health center, noted that a client's failure to take her antihypertensive medication began at the time of the death of a close friend. Miss N. consulted the literature on loss and grieving to gain insight into the significance of this behavior. She also discussed the situation with the social worker, who suggested that the friend may have been helping the client to purchase the medication. This information enabled the nurse to clarify the significance of the relationship with the client and to use what she had learned as the basis for a nursing diagnosis.

It may be necessary to consult references or resource persons during and after the collection of data. It is an important means of ensuring that the assessment is not misdirected or the data misinterpreted. It also helps to reveal the *significance* of assessment findings and to give direction to the *future gathering of data.*

Many nurses postpone consulting the literature until they have struggled over the identification of alterations, thinking that they must have a diagnosis before reading about the alteration. This is a misconception. By consulting books, periodicals, and other reference sources before formulating diagnoses, the nurse will find that her diagnoses will probably be more accurate and easier to formulate.

The findings of assessment will serve as a starting point for use of the literature. Reading about physical, functional, and behavioral areas affected by the client's change in health status helps to explain the significance of assessment data, as does reading about medical diagnoses, signs and symptoms, treatments, medications, and laboratory data.

The nurse can compare her findings in the physiological, psychological, social, cultural, and developmental areas with those that are considered "normal" or "expected" so that she can identify changes in the adaptive status of the client. She will also be better prepared to anticipate *potential* alterations of adaptation and to understand the *nursing* focus of alterations that have already been identified.

To clarify the extent to which adaptive responses to alterations of health status are inadequate, excessive, deficient, or dysfunctional and to put these alterations in order of priority, the nurse can measure or judge the responses in terms of the effect or the potential effect for the client. She may ask:

- Is life threatened?
- Is integrity in any of the dimensions (physiological, psychological, social, cultural, or developmental) at risk?
- Is function in any of the dimensions less than optimal or less than adequate?
- Is the client prevented from achieving his potential?
- Is the client prevented from achieving satisfaction in his life situation?

For every "yes" to the questions just listed, the nurse writes a short descriptive phrase. These phrases, condensed and refined, become part of the nursing diagnoses.

In summary, data that have been obtained as a result of assessment must be evaluated for completeness, correctness, and significance. Knowledge must be used to interpret patterns and relationships within and among the adaptive dimensions. Nursing diagnosis will most often focus on responses to or effects of the altered adaptive status of the client. The alterations of adaptive status that are identified as a result of interpretation and integration of assessment data provide the basis for statements of diagnosis.

STRUCTURE OF THE STATEMENT OF NURSING DIAGNOSIS

It is appropriate here to restate the definition of a nursing diagnosis. *A nursing diagnosis is a statement of a potential or altered health status of a client which is derived from nursing assessment and requires intervention from the domain of nursing.*

Because the practice of stating formal nursing diagnoses is a relatively recent event, no single, precise format is being used by all nurses. The following guidelines are used successfully by many nurses when they formulate nursing diagnoses.

GUIDELINES FOR FORMULATING NURSING DIAGNOSES

1. The diagnostic statement usually consists of two main phrases: the first describes the alteration and the second suggests a basis or reason for the alteration.

2. The "alteration phrase" and the "reason phrase" are connected by an expression of relationship such as "associated with" or "related to."

3. The diagnostic statement should be as concise as possible and expressed in terminology that is generally understood by nurses and other health professionals.

4. Both main phrases of the diagnostic statement should be specific enough to give direction to the remainder of the nursing process.

Use of a suitable connecting expression is very important. There has been a tendency to use the terms "due to" or "caused by" or "as a result of" to connect the main phrases. This is not desirable because these expressions imply a cause and effect relationship that might be difficult to establish with certainty and that might place a legal burden of proof on the nurse who is making the diagnosis (Mundinger and Jauron, 1975).

The relationships described in nursing diagnoses are not always reflective of cause and effect. Assessment data will reveal a probable reason for or factors contributing to the diagnosis, but will not necessarily establish a cause. For this reason it is unwise for the nurse to make statements about causality. Also, the cause of an alteration is not always the factor on which nursing diagnoses and interventions are based. The diagnoses "dizziness caused by altered cerebral circulation" and "risk of injury related to episodes of dizziness" come from the same assessment findings, but the second one states the situation in a way that reflects the nursing focus.

Wording the main phrases as concisely as possible will make it easier to read and record the diagnoses and to include them in the developing classification system. Making the main phrases as specific as possible provides information for all members of the health care team, not just the nurse making the diagnosis, and suggests criteria by which responses to intervention might be evaluated. The diagnosis "impaired home health maintenance related to right-sided paralysis" meets the above guidelines and is specific enough to communicate the nature of the alteration as well as to suggest the direction of intervention.

Use of the above guidelines in most cases results in a nursing diagnosis that communicates the nature of the alteration of adaptive status, suggests a reason or basis for the alteration, and directs the planning of nursing intervention.

VARIATIONS IN STRUCTURE OF THE STATEMENT OF DIAGNOSIS

There will be occasions when the diagnosis cannot be realistically or adequately expressed in a statement that conforms to the guidelines described previously. This can occur in the following situations:

Two alterations are very closely related.
Two or more factors contribute to the alteration.
The basis for the alteration has not yet been established.
The basis for the alteration is too complex to describe in a concise phrase.
The concise statement would be insufficient for the purpose of planning nursing interventions.

When two alterations are so closely related that they require the same planning for intervention, it may be best to state both in the first main phrase of the diagnosis, for example, "anxiety and depression related to marital problems." When two or more factors or reasons contribute to the alteration this may be reflected in the second main phrase, for example, "reduced nutritional intake related to anorexia and poorly fitting dentures."

Occasionally, the diagnostic statement may consist of only the first part. This happens when the presence of the alteration has been established, but the reason or basis for it has not yet been identified, or when the full diagnosis would be difficult to verbalize because of length and complexity. Examples of a "first part only" diagnosis are "reduced function of short-term memory," "frequent falls," "alteration in pattern of sleep — insomnia," and "prolonged mourning." In each of these cases, the reason for the alteration might not yet have been established or might be very complex in nature and would have to be described in a different form.

Because it is not always possible to reconcile the need for clinically useful descriptiveness with the need for conciseness, nursing diagnoses are sometimes organized in levels. When the alteration or potential alteration has many nursing implications, the first level diagnosis might be a very broad statement about the type of alteration or potential alteration. Under this first broad statement of diagnosis might be qualifying diagnoses that are narrower in scope and are more descriptive and specific to the client and to the practice situation. The following is an example:

Physiological and psychological alterations associated with chemotherapy.

- Increased susceptibility to infection related to immunosuppression.
- Disturbance of body image related to loss of scalp and body hair.
- Reduced nutritional intake related to anorexia, nausea, and vomiting.

Another way of fulfilling the requirement for conciseness, while also providing necessary information about the alteration, is to state the diagnosis in a minimum of words and to list briefly assessment findings that support the diagnosis. This has the added advantage of providing additional information from which to form criteria for evaluating responses to intervention. An example of a diagnosis followed by supporting assessment findings follows:

Example: Failure to follow diabetes regimen related to lack of information and under-standing.
Client states she "Used to have diabetes."
Has not refilled prescription for oral hypoglycemic medication.
Requests additional food on tray to "offset weight loss."
Observed ingesting candy bars and other snack foods.

Adding assessment data to support the diagnosis can give valuable insights to the alteration. A nursing student who had diagnosed her client as suffering from a severe change in self-image related to debility and weakness wrote under the diagnosis a statement made to her by the client, "I feel like a worn-out old car."

As each situation presents itself, the nurse has to decide whether the diagnosis can be written within the desired two-part format or whether it is necessary to use one of the alternatives described previously. The decision depends in part on the information available and whether or not the concise format communicates sufficient information upon which to base an accurate plan of care.

In most cases it is desirable to make the diagnosis as narrow and specific as possible. This provides more direction for the setting of goals and the planning of care. For example, the diagnosis "potential for pathological fractures related to severe osteoporosis" is specific and immediately suggests nursing interventions that deal with gentle handling, avoidance of trauma, and reduction of safety hazards. Unfortunately, alterations of adaptive status do not always present themselves in narrow, sharply defined dimensions. Impaired ventilation and alteration in cerebral function are examples of serious alterations that are broad in scope and in nursing implications.

The diagnosis sometimes expresses an event or alteration that *might* occur, rather than one that already exists. This type of situation can be expressed by the use of words such as "potential for" or "risk of"; for example, "risk of digitalis toxicity related to rapid diuresis and reduced level of serum potassium." In this instance, one also recognizes the value of following the diagnosis with pertinent assessment findings — the past 24 hour fluid intake and output volumes as well as the most recent serum potassium level. This is true for most diagnoses describing potential alterations.

In summary, the statement of nursing diagnosis is still an evolving process. For this reason, there is a lack of agreement among nurses about how the statement should be structured. In most cases it is important that the statement be made as specific as possible. The format should be such that it accomplishes a major purpose of diagnosis, that is, to give direction to nursing intervention. The predominant format is a concise statement consisting of a main phrase describing the alteration of adaptive status connected by an expression of relationship such as "related to" or "associated with" to a second main phrase that describes the reason or basis for the alteration. Variations in format may have to be used when the situation is unique or complex or when all of the information needed for formulation of a two-part statement is not available. Diagnoses are written to describe potential alterations of adaptation as well as those that already exist.

PROBLEMS ASSOCIATED WITH STATEMENT OF THE NURSING DIAGNOSIS

Although there are diverse ways of stating the nursing diagnosis, there are some common pitfalls that should be avoided because they affect the accuracy and usefulness of the diagnosis.

A common fallacy of diagnosis is stating the alteration part of the diagnosis in terms of the pathology or the medical diagnosis. Examples of this are the diagnoses "congestive heart failure," "schizophrenia," "fracture of the left femur," and "uterine fibroids." While all of the examples have obvious nursing implications, it is the implications, not the pathology, that should be the foci of the nursing diagnoses. In the case of congestive heart failure, the client could have a nursing diagnosis of "reduced energy level related to decreased oxygenation of tissue." The schizophrenic client might have a diagnosis such as "impairment of communication with others related to suspiciousness and effects of hallucinations." These nursing diagnoses tell something about the *meaning* of the pathology for the client in terms of effects, responses, risks, and disabilities. It is easy to become confused with this aspect of diagnosis because there are some areas of overlap among professions in the use of specific terminology for diagnosis. The diagnosis "depression," for example, may describe pathology to one professional, responses to another.

Care should be taken not to make the diagnosis too general. The diagnosis "risks associated with edema of lower extremities" is too general to be useful because the risks are not named. The second main phrase of a diagnosis also should be as specific as possible. The diagnosis "reduced ability to communicate related to hearing loss" would be much more helpful if the second phrase described concisely the nature and extent of the hearing loss.

Diagnoses should not be written in terms of the client's nursing needs, for example, "client needs help to walk to bathroom." Needs will be identified at many points in the nursing process and will be a consideration in the formulation of the diagnosis and the planning of care, but the statement of diagnosis is broader and, unlike a statement of need, gives information about the reason or basis for the alteration. It is also incorrect to state the nursing diagnosis as a nursing goal or intervention, for example, "client should learn how to give his own insulin" or "reduce safety hazards in the immediate environment." Goals and interventions *result from* the formulation of accurate nursing diagnoses.

In some cases there is a tendency to state the diagnosis in terms of the *nurse's* needs, for example, "dressing change takes 45 minutes." In this diagnosis the focus is inappropriately on the nurse rather than on the client.

The problem of length of time required to change the dressing will be considered when scheduling the dressing change as a part of the plan for care.

Although findings of assessment are the bases for the nursing diagnosis, the assessment findings themselves are not the same as the diagnosis. "Blood pressure is 250/130" and "frequent occipital headaches" are not nursing diagnoses. They are isolated assessment findings that must be considered and interpreted along with other data to arrive at a basis for diagnosis.

Sometimes the main phrases are mistakenly reversed. In the example "lack of knowledge about blood pressure medication related to tendency to omit doses," the main phrases are reversed. Omitting doses of medication is an alteration in health maintenance behavior that is related to the client's lack of knowledge.

Occasionally, both main phrases of the diagnosis say the same thing in different words. "Ulceration of sacral area related to skin breakdown," "decreased thyroid function related to hypothyroidism," and "injury of left wrist related to fracture of the radius" are examples of this.

Stating several unrelated alterations in the same phrase makes it difficult to use the diagnosis in the planning of care even though the etiology of the alterations may be the same. Examples are "lesion of left foot and reduced vision related to vascular changes of diabetes mellitus" and "reduced level of activity and depression related to episodes of angina pectoris." When alterations are unrelated, as they are above, they will usually require separate plans for intervention, which is more easily accomplished if each alteration is described in a separate diagnosis.

The nurse should resist the temptation to write the diagnosis in such elegant terms that the meaning is not clear to everyone who will need to use it. "Compromised integrity of the integument" is an accurate phrase, but may not communicate to all persons working with a client that skin breakdown has occurred. Overuse of specialized jargon and abbreviations is to be avoided, too, since it may make the diagnosis less clear to others. Terms such as "stroking out" for cerebrovascular accident or stroke and "G.I. bleed" when gastrointestinal hemorrhage is meant can confuse the issue for someone not familiar with this jargon. Abbreviations that are not standard across the health care professions are also confusing.

The statement of nursing diagnosis should not contain value-laden terms or judgmental expressions. Words like "demanding," "uncooperative," or "complaining" should not be used, since they are usually the result of subjective rather than objective interpretations of behavior and tend to label the client. Negative judgments about care given by health workers are, of course, a matter of concern to the nurse but have strong legal implications when included in a nursing diagnosis. For this reason, "anxiety related to the physician not explaining the diagnosis" might be better stated as "anxiety related to lack of information about the medical diagnosis Crohn's disease." Another example, "potential for contractures of extremities related to incorrect positioning," might be better stated as related to "lack of alignment."

At times, a diagnosis may reflect a state that should not or cannot be corrected by nursing intervention. "Grieving related to recent death of spouse" describes a process that should not be interrupted. Of course, there are other implications concerning the client's loss about which diagnoses can be written and care plans formulated. The diagnosis "inability to see related to severe retinopathy" describes a state that cannot be corrected by nursing intervention. Nursing diagnoses in this case would be properly directed toward the best possible level of adaptation by the client to this sensory deficit.

Nurses should be certain that the nursing diagnoses they have made are supported by assessment data and are not based solely on their expectations. Pain is not always the major problem with postoperative or cancer patients, and not every person with a medical diagnosis of congestive heart failue is experiencing shortness of breath. Caution should also be exercised to assure that diagnosis of a potential alteration is realistic. For example, potential for infection is almost constantly present in the person with an indwelling urinary catheter, but potential for infection in the postoperative patient depends on many factors: extent of trauma, type of surgery, number of days since surgery, general health of the person, and others.

The statement of nursing diagnosis should reflect the collaborative nature of the nurse-client relationship. For this reason, terms such as "non-compliance," which are often used by health professionals to describe client behavior related to the health regimen and which suggest a yielding or passive role for the client, should not be used in the diagnostic statement. There are alternative terms such as "adherence" or "maintenance" that are more reflective of the autonomy of the client in relation to his health behavior.

Finally, it is necessary to discuss failure to write the diagnosis at all. When this happens, it is usually because the nurse cannot figure out how to write the diagnosis. Familiar is the plea, "I know this is a problem, but I just don't know how to write it." The best advice for the nurse in this predicament is to write the diagnosis in the best way possible, making sure that all significant points are written accurately and in a manner that can be understood by all.

CHANGING THE DIAGNOSIS

The sense of accomplishment experienced by the nurse who has produced a neatly phrased nursing diagnosis may be short-lived, for the nursing diagnosis, by its very nature, is not a permanent thing. In some cases the goals of intervention will be accomplished and no more work with a specific diagnosis will be required; in others, an old diagnosis must be replaced by a new one. In many cases, however, ongoing nursing assessment reveals that a diagnosis has to be revised because of changes in the client or the situation. When an existing diagnosis is changed, the focus of it may remain the same, but either phrase (occasionally both) may have to be revised. This is necessary when

- New data have emerged.
- The client's level of adaptation or position on the health-illness continuum has changed.
- The priority focus of the diagnosis has changed.

Acquisition of significant new data is the most frequent reason for a change in the diagnosis, since it often results in new insights into the alteration or factors contributing to the alteration. A diagnosis initially stated as "failure to continue anti-hypertensive medication related to lack of understanding of hypertension" may become "reluctance to continue anti-hypertensive medication related to experience of the side effect, impotence."

Change in the *level of adaptation* or *position on the health-illness continuum* requires revision of the diagnosis. The diagnosis "reduced ability to carry out the activities of daily living related to decreased energy level," may change in either direction to "inability to carry out the activities of daily living related to severe weakness" or to "reduced ability to carry out strenuous activities related to limited energy reserve." Of course the care plan will change with the diagnosis.

When the *priority focus* of the diagnosis changes, the diagnosis may need to be reworded. The client's response to the surgical creation of a stoma may change as he progresses through the stages of crisis and begins to incorporate the stoma into his body image. Nursing intervention must be adapted to the different stages in the client's response. The first stage may be related to the trauma of surgery, the next stage to the presence of the stoma itself and the loss of normal patterns of elimination, and a later stage to the need to understand how this alteration can be made to become less disruptive to his style of living. The wording of the diagnosis will need to reflect the current status of the response.

USE OF PUBLISHED NURSING DIAGNOSES

There are several publications available to the nurse in which diagnoses commonly found in nursing are categorized and listed with assessment findings relevant to each diagnosis (Campbell, 1978; Gebbie, 1976; Gebbie and Lavin, 1975). The general nursing literature also reflects the growing use of nursing diagnosis; recent textbooks and periodicals frequently contain examples of nursing diagnoses related to the topic being discussed.

There are advantages and disadvantages to the use of already formulated diagnoses. Major advantages include the fact that they offer to the nurse access to a wide variety of correctly stated diagnoses, and provide the opportunity to validate individual judgments about alterations within the domain of nursing. Published diagnoses are also written in a way that carefully communicate the nursing focus. Disadvantages include the fact that a published diagnosis is not tailored to the specific client or situation and for that reason may require one or more qualifying diagnoses. Also, many types of diagnostic statements are not yet in the literature, and the ones that have been published are not always written with consistent guidelines. However, if properly used, published diagnoses can be a valuable addition to the nurse's own efforts in the formulation of nursing diagnoses.

SUMMARY

Designation of nursing diagnosis as a separate and distinct step of the nursing process is a relatively recent event. For this reason, there is a lack of uniformity in the way nurses approach this step. The two major requirements for successful nursing diagnosis are an accurate and thorough nursing assessment and the judicious use of nursing and related knowledge throughout the diagnostic process.

To be useful for diagnosis, data collection during assessment must be as accurate and complete as possible, and all sources of information must be utilized. Sources of assessment data include interviews with the client or family or both, use of the skills of observation and examination, thorough review of laboratory data and health records, consultation with nursing and other health care professionals, and use of the literature of nursing and related disciplines. The nurse organizes the collection and recording of data in a systematic way by use of an assessment form and adjusts the process to the requirements of the situation, the setting, and the purpose for which the client is seeking health care as well as to the uniqueness of the client himself.

When formulating the diagnosis, the nurse will integrate and interpret the assessment data in a way that facilitates the identification of alterations of adaptation experienced by the client, with attention to the effects and responses resulting from change in health status. The statement of nursing diagnosis ideally consists of two parts: The first part describes the alteration of adaptive status that the client is experiencing; the second part identifies the basis or reason for the alteration. The parts are joined by an expression of relationship such as "associated with" or "related to." The diagnosis should be stated in a way that expresses the nursing focus and gives direction to the rest of the nursing process. Although concisely written, the diagnosis should be specific enough to be useful and should employ terminology that communicates accurately to all nurses and other health professionals.

The nurse approaching the task of stating a nursing diagnosis should decide what information needs to be communicated and should then follow, as closely as possible, the guidelines that have been presented in this chapter. In nursing diagnosis, as in many things, practice makes perfect.

References

Campbell, C.: *Nursing diagnosis and intervention in nursing practice.* New York, John Wiley & Sons, 1978.

Gebbie, K.M. (ed): *Classification of nursing diagnoses — Summary of the second national conference.* St. Louis, The Clearinghouse — National Group for Classification of Nursing Diagnoses, 1976.

Gebbie, K.M., and Lavin, M.A. (eds.): *Classification of nursing diagnoses — Proceedings of the first national conference.* St. Louis, The C.V. Mosby Company, 1975.

Mundinger, M.O., and Jauron, G.D.: Developing a nursing diagnosis. *Nursing Outlook,* 23:94, 1975.

Webster's Third New International Dictionary of the English Language. Unabridged. Springfield, Mass., G. & C. Merriam Company, 1976.

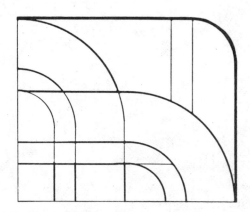

SECTION TWO

NURSING DIAGNOSIS:

Realities of Utilization

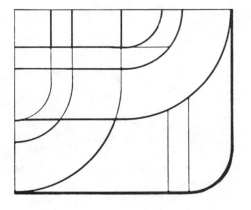

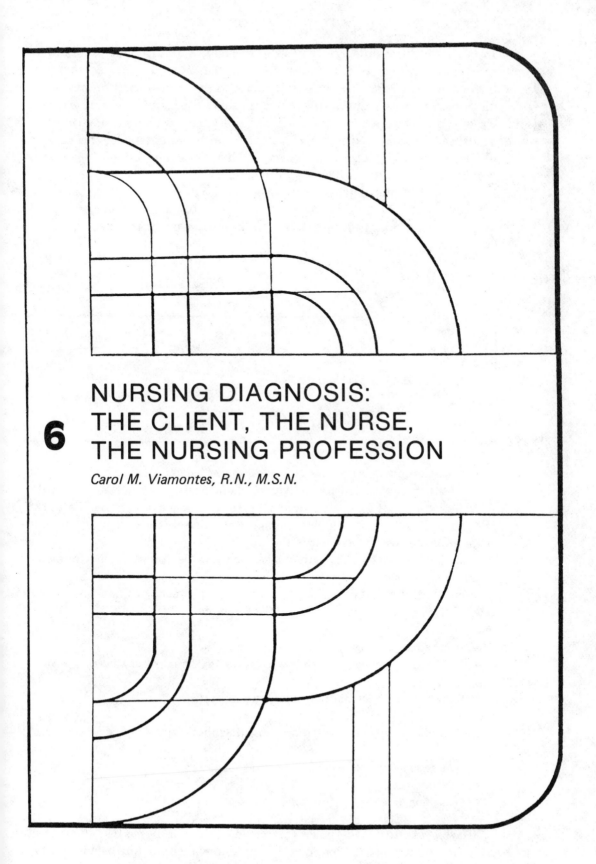

NURSING DIAGNOSIS:
THE CLIENT, THE NURSE,
THE NURSING PROFESSION

6

Carol M. Viamontes, R.N., M.S.N.

In order to utilize nursing diagnosis effectively, the nurse must be aware of the advantages and difficulties that accompany its use. A thorough understanding of the practicalities involved in the implementation of nursing diagnosis can play a crucial role in maximizing benefits and devising effective ways to deal with nursing problems. The practical and theoretical advantages of properly formulated nursing diagnoses can be considerable; this chapter discusses these advantages in terms of their influence on the client, the individual nurse, and the nursing profession.

The use of nursing diagnosis is not without its difficulties, but these difficulties can be minimized over a period of time by increasing the knowledge and skills necessary to engage in the diagnostic process.

THE CLIENT AND NURSING DIAGNOSIS

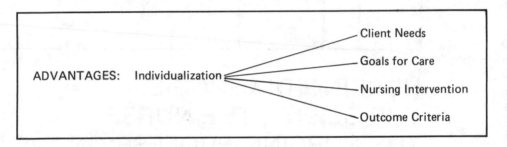

The use of nursing diagnosis provides major advantages to the client. It enables the nurse to identify individual client health care needs, aids in the formulation of specific goals attainable through nursing action, facilitates the selection of appropriate nursing therapies, and directs the design of outcome criteria for purposes of evaluation.

An illustration of this individualization can be found in the following example:

Mr. Vincent is admitted to the hospital with a medical diagnosis of renal calculi. Nursing diagnoses for this patient include:

- Impaired urinary elimination related to renal calculi
- Right-sided flank pain related to increased hydrostatic pressure in renal pelvis and ureter
- Risk of urinary tract infection related to urinary stasis

Goals for nursing care based on these diagnoses include:

- Restoration of urinary elimination pattern
- Resolution of pain
- Prevention of urinary tract infection

Having identified the goals for nursing care, the nurse can then select appropriate nursing interventions that are individualized for the client. Here are some examples of nursing interventions in the case of Mr. Vincent:

- Monitor intake and output.
- Force fluids to 3000 cc/day
- Administer prescribed meperidine 50 mg every 3 hours during periods of renal colic.
- Instruct patient on acid-ash diet.

Once goals for nursing care have been established, criteria for the evaluation of nursing care can likewise be determined; both goals and outcome criteria evolve from the statement of client-specific nursing diagnoses. Outcome criteria for Mr. Vincent would include:

- Intake is equal to output
- Absence of right-sided flank pain
- Negative urine culture
- Urinary pH <5.5

The use of nursing diagnosis aids the nurse in identifying a wide spectrum of actual and potential health care needs. It enhances the quality of patient care by focusing it in terms of a series of well-defined goals that are client-specific. Thus, nursing diagnosis guides the planning and implementation of specific nursing therapies and facilitates the identification of outcome criteria necessary for the evaluation of nursing care.

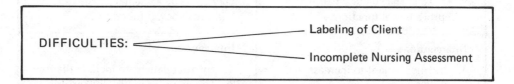

DIFFICULTIES: — Labeling of Client
— Incomplete Nursing Assessment

Certain serious but preventable difficulties may arise from the use of nursing diagnosis. One major problem with a system that involves labeling and classification is that the nurse may tend to put clients into predetermined diagnostic categories rather than formulate specific diagnoses based on an individualized nursing assessment. The client is thus "labeled," and, instead of being treated as a unique individual, he or she becomes part of a group with predetermined characteristics. When this happens, a loss of identity can occur, and the client may be referred to as "the R-sided flank pain in Room 349."

A second difficulty that usually stems from the first is an incomplete nursing assessment. The nursing assessment may be incomplete because the nurse has already labeled the client and therefore does not take the time to listen, observe carefully, and formulate a complete list of nursing diagnoses. The remaining sequence of steps in the nursing process, that is, planning, intervention, and evaluation, is therefore liable to be inappropriate in meeting the health care needs of the client. A clinical example will clarify these points.

Two hospitalized patients, Mr. Jones and Mr. Wolf, have the following nursing diagnosis: *"constipation related to irregular dietary habits."* For both of these patients, a change in dietary patterns is an appropriate plan of care. With no further assessment data other than those related to this nursing diagnosis, it would follow that these patients should be instructed concerning a high-fiber diet. However, when the nurse carries out a more in-depth assessment, she discovers that Mr. Jones dislikes many high-fiber foods, and Mr. Wolf needs to maintain a restricted caloric diet because of diabetes mellitus. As a result, the diets as well as instructions to these patients must be different. Figure 6–1 illustrates the individualized care plans for these two clients in relation to this nursing diagnosis.

The previous example illustrates that if the nurse had implemented duplicate care plans for both patients, the resulting care for one of the patients would have been inappropriate and ineffective. One must keep in mind that nursing diagnoses must be individualized for each client. Assessments must

Patient: Mr. Jones (history of arteriosclerotic heart disease).	Patient: Mr. Wolf (history of diabetes mellitus).
Nursing Diagnosis: Constipation related to irregular dietary habits.	**Nursing Diagnosis:** Constipation related to irregular dietary habits.
Plan: To change dietary habits to improve bowel function.	**Plan:** To change dietary habits to improve bowel function.

Intervention:
 	
1. Instruct patient to increase fluid intake:
    1 glass of tea or fruit juice between meals.
    1 glass of prune juice at breakfast.
 	
2. Instruct patient to increase intake of natural laxative foods:
    dried prunes or figs as a bedtime snack.
	Intervention:
	
	1. Instruct patient to include the following foods in his 1800 calorie ADA diet:
	    ½ cup bran cereal = 1 bread exchange
	    lettuce salad with 1 teaspoon French dressing = 1 fat exchange
	    2 medium prunes = 1 fruit exchange
	    1 medium fig = 1 fruit exchange.
	
	2. Instruct patient to increase daily fluid intake with the following "free" foods:
	    coffee, tea, unsweetened cranberry juice, mixed vegetable juice, tomato juice.

Evaluation: **Outcome Criteria:** Decreased incidence of constipation.	Evaluation: **Outcome Criteria:** Decreased incidence of constipation.

Figure 6–1 Examples of individualized care plans.

be complete before nursing diagnoses can be stated and before nursing care plans can be developed. The nurse must recognize that, although people have many aspects in common, every individual is unique and must be treated as such.

THE NURSE AND NURSING DIAGNOSIS

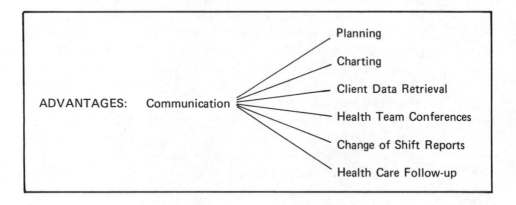

The use of nursing diagnosis offers a number of advantages to the individual nurse, particularly in the area of communication. Most health care settings feature interactions among members of a team, and nursing diagnoses can function to improve communication as well as planning between individual nurses, nurses and physicians, and nurses and various allied health professionals. Much of this improved communication results from the use of well-defined, standardized terminology to identify and discuss health care needs as well as develop plans of care. Other areas in which nursing diagnoses enhance communication include nursing care plans, charting, client data retrieval, change of shift reports, and discharge planning.

In *nursing care plans*, nursing diagnoses provide crucial information about the health care needs that have been identified. Nurses not familiar with a client can refer to his care plan and be able to determine very specifically his primary and secondary needs. Other health professionals, such as physical therapists, social workers, and dietitians, can refer to nursing diagnoses previously identified when planning appropriate therapies. For example, Ms. Smith, a dietitian, was requested to see Mr. Schneider, a diabetic at a neighborhood health center. His diabetes mellitus was uncontrolled because he was not adhering to an 1800 calorie ADA diet. Before talking with Mr. Schneider, Ms. Smith referred to the nursing care plan that had been developed by his primary nurse. She noted the following nursing diagnoses:

1. Non-adherence to dietary regimen related to cultural dietary habits (Germanic).

2. Lack of understanding of diet therapy related to a language barrier.

Based on this information, Ms. Smith was able to plan a diet incorporating various German dishes. She also discovered that Mr. Schneider's brother spoke English well. She talked to him and he agreed to help his brother plan meals.

A second advantage to the nurse in utilizing nursing diagnosis is in *charting*, particularly when the problem-oriented record is used to document information about clients. This type of integrated record system is oriented to client problems and can be utilized by all health team members. Nurses, physicians, and allied health professionals list their diagnoses on the client's record, indicating the chronological order in which the diagnoses are made (Fig. 6–2). When changes in the client's health status occur, the appropriate diagnosis as well as assessment data and plans are recorded in progress notes (Fig. 6–3). The use of nursing diagnosis in this record system allows for the presentation of large amounts of information synthesized into a statement or label. Thus, this information can be easily understood and can be used in treatment planning.

A third advantage to the nurse is the possibility of *client data retrieval* based on identified nursing diagnoses. At present, this is not entirely feasible because a standardized taxonomy of nursing diagnoses has not been fully developed; once this classification process is complete and accepted as a

Client: Mr. A. Hoffman, a 49 year old male. Admitted 9/20 with complaints of shortness of breath on exertion and a productive cough.

Date	Number	Diagnosis
9/20	1	Chronic obstructive lung disease.
		S. Jones, M.D.
9/20	2	Restriction in mobility related to shortness of breath on exertion.
		M. Wilson, R.N.
9/20	3	Alteration in self-concept related to inability to participate in sports.
		M. Wilson, R.N.
9/20	4	Impaired ventilation, related to COPD.
		D. Frank, R.R.T.
9/20	5	Risk of lung cancer, related to three packs per day smoking habit.
		M. Wilson, R.N., and D. Frank, R.R.T.
9/21	6	Increased level of anxiety related to effect of withdrawal from smoking.
		M. Wilson, R.N.

Figure 6-2 Sample list of diagnoses.

Date	Diagnosis	Notes
9/21 8 a.m.	1	COPD. Temp. 101.2°F. Sputum is purulent. Get sputum for C&S. Bedrest. ASA gr X q 4 hr for temp. 100°F. IPPB with Mucomyst q 4 hr. O_2 per nasal cannula 2 L/min. *S. Jones, M.D.*
9/21 10 a.m.	4	Impaired ventilation. Skin appears dusky. Wheezing noted. IPPB treatment administered. Expectorated large amount of purulent sputum. Suggest chest physiotherapy and adding Bronkosol to IPPB treatments. *D. Frank, R.R.T.*
9/21 1 p.m.	6	Increased anxiety. Increasing restlessness. Verbalizing desire to smoke. Threatens to leave hospital A.M.A. Suggest allowing patient to smoke one cigarette per shift, with O_2 off. *M. Wilson, R.N.*

Figure 6–3 Sample progress notes from problem-oriented record of patient in Figure 6-2.

useful informational system, data retrieval based on nursing diagnosis will be accomplished with the ease that now accompanies retrieval based on medical diagnosis. Such a data base will prove a rich resource in the development of nursing's unique body of knowledge.

A fourth advantage to the nurse is the facilitation of communication in *health team conferences*. In this setting, nursing diagnoses are useful in organizing discussions regarding health care strategies for individual clients. For example, one nursing team conference focused on a 45 year old male client with a compound fracture of the femur. In addition to the obvious nursing diagnosis of *restricted mobility and pain related to the compound fracture*, this client also had a *moderate anxiety related to the loss of income and possible loss of his job*. Identification of the latter diagnosis resulted in inviting a social worker to the next team conference to share her expertise in planning appropriate therapies for the reduction of the client's anxiety.

A fifth advantage of nursing diagnosis is the improvement in *change of shift reports*. Many such reports are lengthy and often contain disorganized information. They can be made more concise by classifying changes in the client's health status under specific nursing diagnoses that have been formulated. As new nursing diagnoses are identified, they can be added to the nursing reports. For example, Mr. Carl, a 69 year old patient with a cerebral vascular accident, had a *risk of skin breakdown on his coccyx related to immobility*. He also had numerous other nursing diagnoses, but his risk for skin breakdown was a priority. At the end of the day shift, the nurse reported that there was a reddened area 1 cm by 2 cm on his coccyx, and it had a raw appearance. At this time, the nursing diagnosis was changed to *"decubitus ulcer related to restricted mobilization."* The nurses did not have to report on other aspects of Mr. Carl's health status because these were stable. Thus, attention was focused on a priority health care need and appropriate nursing therapies planned and implemented.

A sixth advantage is that the use of nursing diagnosis in the hospital setting can facilitate *community health care follow-up* when the patient returns home. Community health nurses review hospital records in order to determine the health status of the client prior to his return home. A list of nursing diagnoses tells the community health nurse what the client's needs were during his hospitalization and provides a basis for determining what the client's health needs are at present. The following example shows this point more clearly:

A client was admitted to the hospital with uncontrolled diabetes mellitus. During the assessment, the nurse discovered that the client had not been taking his oral hypoglycemics, had not followed the prescribed 1600 calorie ADA diet, and had not given himself proper foot care. The following nursing diagnoses were developed:

1. Non-adherence to prescribed drug therapy related to lack of understanding of disease process.

2. Non-adherence to prescribed diet therapy related to lack of knowledge of diet restriction.

The nursing staff identified some short- and long-term goals and developed a teaching plan for the client and his family. In implementing the nursing care plan, the staff discovered some communication problems between the client and his family that contributed to his non-adherence to medical treatments. An additional nursing diagnosis was made, based on new data that had been collected: *Failure to communicate related to hostility among family members.* When the client was discharged from the hospital, a referral was made to the Visiting Nurse Association. Because the nursing diagnoses had been stated so clearly during the hospitalization, the visiting nurse was able to quickly evaluate the client and his family and make a subsequent referral to a counselor who could work on the communication problems.

As the previous example illustrates, the benefits of nursing diagnosis for the individual nurse are considerable. In summary, they provide information about a client's health needs and enhance communication and planning among the various health care professionals. Further, they improve charting of nurses' notes, facilitate health team conferences and team reports, and promote continuity of care between the health care setting and home.

DIFFICULTIES: — Limited Knowledge / Undeveloped Taxonomy

There are a number of difficulties that individual nurses have encountered in utilizing nursing diagnoses. One is that many nurses have limited knowledge of the concepts of the nursing process and nursing diagnosis. Educational institutions vary in their approach to the teaching of nursing. The concept of nursing process may or may not be utilized, and the components of that process are not necessarily defined in the same manner by all. Nursing diagnosis, as a part of that process, has only recently received any widespread attention. As a distinct entity of nursing practice, diagnosis is only now being defined, and knowledge of its meaning and application is still limited. Of those nurses who have heard the term "nursing diagnosis," many are unfamiliar with the steps in formulating diagnoses and, hence, tend to use them inappropriately or not at all. The general consequence of these educational and historical factors is a significant population of nurses who are neither educated about nor committed to the use of nursing diagnosis.

Resources do exist for correcting these deficiencies; texts such as this, curricular changes at the basic and continuing education levels, and increasing development of the knowledge and uses of nursing diagnosis are but a few general approaches to correcting present deficiencies.

For the individual nurse who desires to increase her knowledge of nursing diagnosis, the following resources are available:

- Lists of nursing diagnoses developed at the four National Conferences can be obtained from the Clearinghouse for the Classification of Nursing Diagnosis.
- Local, state, and regional nursing diagnosis conferences are being conducted and are open to any nurse interested in and working with nursing diagnosis.
- Nursing Diagnosis Newsletter (Nr. Dx.), the official newsletter for the National Group for the Classification of Nursing Diagnosis, provides updated information on recent developments in nursing diagnosis in the areas of nursing education, practice, and research.
- Recent nursing literature increasingly includes nursing diagnosis as a topic.
- Annotated bibliographies have been compiled by various nursing groups across the country and are available through the Clearinghouse for the Classification of Nursing Diagnosis.

Another difficulty for the nurse is the lack of a sophisticated taxonomy of diagnostic labels. One of the specific purposes for the initiation of the National Conferences was to begin the development of a taxonomy. Many diagnoses have already been identified and tentatively organized into appropriate categories. A system for classification that includes signs and symptoms appropriate to the various diagnostic categories is currently being developed.

All of these difficulties contribute to a general feeling of frustration on the part of those nurses attempting to learn about and utilize nursing diagnoses. General knowledge of nursing diagnosis is limited at present mainly because standardization and dissemination of the process are still in early stages, and only limited numbers of nurses are involved in the development of the conceptual framework and basic taxonomy by which nursing diagnoses should be formulated. However, work is progressing that should remedy these difficulties. Local and regional conferences that are held on a regular basis devote time to the development of nursing diagnoses and to the discussion of utilization of nursing diagnoses in various health care settings. Results of these conferences are presented at biennial national conferences and published in *Nr. Dx.*

THE NURSING PROFESSION AND NURSING DIAGNOSIS

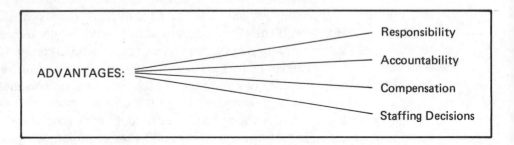

In addition to the benefits of nursing diagnosis for the client and the individual nurse, there are also important advantages for the nursing profession as a whole. The first advantage is that the use of nursing diagnosis helps define the domain of nursing to health care administrators, legislators, and other health care providers and consumers. In the past, these groups have lacked a clear and unified understanding of the role, functions, and responsibilities of nursing. The use of nursing diagnosis has helped to change this situation.

Demands for accountability increase when areas of responsibility are clearly identified. Today, such demands are increasingly voiced by the public and the professions, who claim that nurses should be responsible and accountable for the care they deliver.

In order to determine the quality of nursing care being given, a variety of ongoing quality assurance programs have been developed. The purposes of these programs are:

1. To determine by objective measurements the effectiveness of nursing care being provided to clients

2. To implement changes in nursing care based on information obtained from these measurements

Nursing diagnoses can be extremely valuable in determing the effectiveness of the health care that is being provided by nurses. For example, nursing diagnoses can facilitate nursing audits, an important means by which nursing care is evaluated. In an audit, specific measurable criteria are identified for each type of nursing care provided. Health records are then examined to determine if the care provided to a client was appropriate and effective. Nursing diagnoses facilitate the auditing process by serving to identify problem areas.

A third advantage to the nursing profession is that nursing diagnoses can be used to validate services provided by nurses. This is particularly important in terms of third party payments. Nursing diagnoses help in identifying which nursing functions are independent, which are interdependent, and which are dependent upon other health professionals. At present, insurance companies in many states reimburse only those services provided according to the medical diagnoses identified for each client. Nursing services are reimbursed only when ordered by a physician or when executed under a physician's supervision. This policy creates two problems. The first is that many clients who do not have access to medical care are not able to utilize available nursing care, for example, in clinics, because their health insurance does not cover nursing services. The second problem is that nurses are not able to deliver nursing care unless a physician determines its need or supervises the care. In some states, however, nurse practice acts have specifically defined the independent functions of a nurse, and some nurse practitioners are beginning to receive reimbursement for services provided. These nurse practitioners have utilized individual nursing diagnoses to delineate the domain of their independent nursing functions. When a sophisticated classification system of nursing diagnoses exists, the nursing profession will be able to clearly define all independent nursing functions to third party payers. More importantly, clients who have had limited access to health care in the past will then be able to utilize available care provided by nurse practitioners.

The fourth advantage that nursing diagnosis provides to the nursing profession is that it facilitates staffing patterns, which can be helpful to nursing service departments. By examining the nursing diagnoses that have been identified for a particular group of patients, a nursing service administrator can determine needs for specific nursing functions in that patient care area. For example, one clinical nurse specialist observed that, in a group of diabetic patients on a general medical unit, the following nursing diagnoses were prevalent:

1. Absence of interest in present health state

2. Lack of knowledge of diet therapy

3. Lack of knowledge of drug therapy

4. Non-compliance with preventive health measures related to inappropriate perception of disease condition

Based on this information, the nurse requested that a patient health educator be assigned to the unit to develop, implement, and evaluate a patient education program for this group of diabetic patients.

```
┌──────────────────────────────────────────────────────────────────┐
│                                   ─── Inter-Professional Misunderstanding │
│  DIFFICULTIES:  ─────────────<                                      │
│                                   ─── Intra-Professional Confusion   │
└──────────────────────────────────────────────────────────────────┘
```

A major problem that affects the nursing profession as a whole is that many health professionals, particularly physicians, question the meaning and implications of nursing diagnosis. They do not believe that nursing diagnoses are an integral part of health care. They have seen the act of diagnosing as being solely a medical function and question whether nurses should actually diagnose. The conflict centers on the word "diagnose." This problem can be attributed to a lack of understanding of the concept of nursing diagnosis. The solution lies in improving communication with health care professionals regarding the concept of nursing diagnosis and in educating them in how nurses formulate and use diagnoses. Other professionals need to be shown the advantages to their practice when nursing diagnoses are used.

Another difficulty for the profession is the lack of agreement among groups of nurses regarding the nature of nursing diagnosis. There are differences of opinion about how diagnoses should be formulated and how terminology should be used. This lack of agreement contributes to a communication problem between those attempting to teach the concepts of nursing diagnosis and those attempting to learn them. Nurses exposed to nursing diagnosis for the first time often become confused and have difficulty committing themselves to this concept when they realize that nursing leaders can't even agree on such fundamental principles as a conceptual framework and a standard taxonomy. In addition to this, there is a continued emphasis placed on disease models rather than health models in formulating nursing diagnoses. Thus, although the nursing profession is striving to promote health and to deal with wellness in addition to illness, some nurses have difficulty accepting the holistic nature of nursing diagnosis because their educational background focused primarily on disease. This problem can be resolved when a standard classification system has been developed and when all schools of nursing revise curricula to reflect health models.

As has been discussed previously, there are considerable benefits, as well as a number of difficulties, inherent in the use of nursing diagnosis. Because nursing diagnosis is in an evolving state, many of the difficulties that have been identified should be partially or completely eliminated in the future.

SUMMARY

This chapter has discussed the realities of utilizing nursing diagnoses for the client, the nurse, and the nursing profession. When properly formulated and implemented, nursing diagnoses can provide an excellent conceptual and practical base for patient care. Conceptually, it provides a holistic orientation that should promote identification of all of the problems of the individual patient. In addition, its emphasis on wellness as well as disease extends its usefulness beyond the immediate treatment of illness and makes it a valuable tool in encouraging practices that will promote health. Patient teaching in acute care and community health settings is one specific area in which these considerations gain major importance.

Practically, nursing diagnoses are extremely useful for the planning, coordination, implementation, and evaluation of health care. In settings where more than one nurse is involved in the care of an individual patient, nursing diagnoses can provide coherence and continuity to patient care. In addition, in settings where a health team is involved, nursing diagnoses can provide a sound base on which therapeutic strategies can be developed.

The above discussion of difficulties, however, underscores the need for coherence and agreement on the basic nature and terminology of nursing diagnoses, since the facilitation of communication is one of the major benefits of this process. At least at a local level, the decision to use nursing diagnoses should be followed by some standardization of their form.

An extremely important factor that will play a crucial role in the future of nursing diagnosis is education. Acceptance of this process will be contingent on making all members of the nursing and other health professions aware of its benefits and willing to work to overcome its difficulties, which are mainly related to communication and standardization.

Above all, however, the ultimate success or failure of the development and utilization of nursing diagnoses will rest with the individual nurse. Commitment to the use of nursing diagnosis is the single most important factor that will determine whether this step in the nursing process will be accepted and implemented universally. Commitment to improved quality of care and the belief that the use of nursing diagnosis will improve that quality should provide the needed incentives to overcome the short-term obstacles initially encountered.

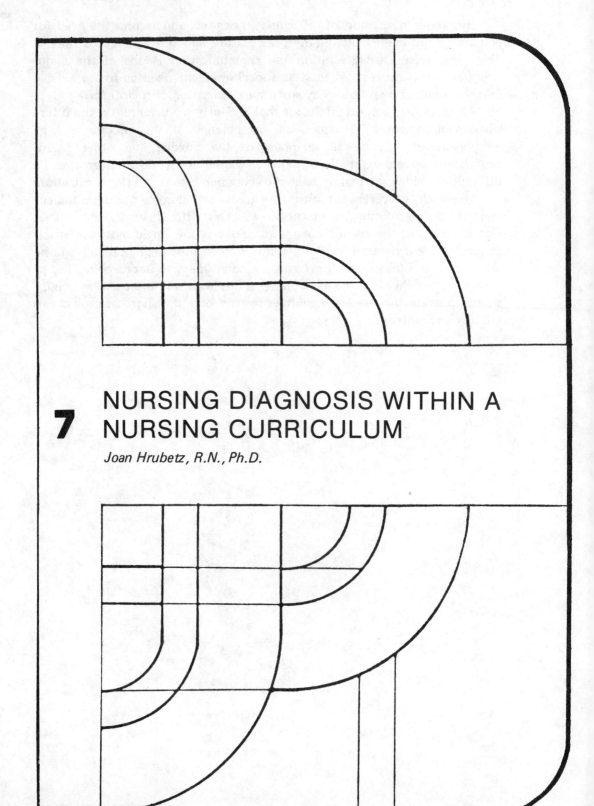

7 NURSING DIAGNOSIS WITHIN A NURSING CURRICULUM

Joan Hrubetz, R.N., Ph.D.

Nursing educators involved in curriculum development have a weighty task. They must prepare today the professional nurse of tomorrow. The nurse of the future cannot be educated in a curriculum that does not take into account those issues with which nursing is currently struggling. These issues are many and include theories of nursing, scope of practice, accountability, and nursing diagnosis. Only one of these issues, *nursing diagnosis*, is relevant here.

Curriculum development is, by its very nature, a dynamic process. In spite of the observable trends in nursing, educators in the nursing field are making decisions based on predictions rather than actual knowledge of the future. On the other hand, they are helping to shape that future by preparing those who will be practicing in it. It is the responsibility, then, of nursing education to prepare nurses with knowledge and skills that can enable them to practice and to lay a foundation for acquisition of knowledge and skills beyond those needed for the predictable future.

Nursing process, the structure for nursing practice, is utilized in nursing curricula as the foundation upon which nursing courses are built. The nursing process is the identification and meeting of client needs that are not technical and are unrelated to doctors' orders (Roy, 1975). The first step of this process, *assessment*, is, without question, not only the responsibility of nurses, but fundamental to their practice. Nurses since Nightingale have been observers, and although the scope of their observations has widened, assessment remains the basic vehicle upon which all their actions are based. The second step of the nursing process, *nursing diagnosis*, however, is not so clearly accepted or widespread among those responsible for preparing nurses for practice. Traditionally, this second step has been labeled "patient problem." As such, nurses have searched out, during their client assessments, everything from physical limitations to sociological implications stemming from a pathological condition. Nursing instructors have been known to tell students that, since all clients are individuals, no two patient health problems should be alike. If this were analogous to the medical model, the logical result would be that no two clients could have the same medical problem! Of course, this is absurd and is used here only to dramatize a point. Aspinall (1976) speculated that nurses ". . . seemed not to understand the relationship of certain signs and symptoms to problem entities. Thus, a nurse would list pulmonary embolus as a possible problem, but she would also list as separate problems the signs and symptoms of pulmonary embolus, such as dyspnea, CO_2 narcosis, and respiratory embarrassment." *Nursing diagnosis does not require signs and symptoms of a medical diagnosis but, by definition, a statement of a potential or actual altered health status of a client(s), which is derived from nursing assessment and requires intervention from the domain of nursing.* Therefore, in Aspinall's example, pulmonary embolus would not be a client problem requiring nursing intervention for amelioration. Rather, the nurse would assess the client's status based upon her observations of the way in which the medical diagnosis of pulmonary embolus affects the client's state of health or illness. Thus, a nursing diagnosis concomitant with the medical diagnosis, pulmonary embolus, might be *"anxiety related to respiratory distress."*

The implications for curriculum development are clear. One of the outcomes of the First National Conference on the Classification of Nursing Diagnosis was a statement on nursing education: The primary professional goal of nursing education should be the communication of relevant nursing knowledge to nursing students. This, obviously, is not a revolutionary insight, but in light of current trends in nursing practice, it represents the necessity for *nursing diagnosis to be an integral part of a nursing curriculum.*

The curriculum development process is a well-known one and can be expressed by a flow chart.

Statement of Philosophy

↓

Theoretical Framework

↓

Statements of Terminal Behaviors

↓

Statements of Level Behaviors

↓

Course Objectives

↓

Individual Lecture Objectives

↓

Selection of Clinical Practice Experiences

Like the research process, which includes problem identification, review of literature, hypotheses formulation, data gathering, data analysis, and interpretation of results, the nursing process is not a lock-step one. As in research, curriculum development follows a pattern, but as each step is defined, new information or greater precision may be added to the previous step. For example, after the philosophy is stated and the conceptual framework evolves from this philosophy, an additional statement about the essence of nursing may be added to the philosophy as a result of the research surrounding the developing conceptual framework.

If, in a school's statement of philosophy, nursing diagnosis is identified as a step in the nursing process, this will be reflected in the conceptual framework, regardless of the focus of that framework. A terminal behavior statement resulting from such a philosophy and conceptual framework may read: "Utilizes all steps of the nursing process in a variety of settings." Such a statement is then seen in each of the preceding level objectives. For example, at the completion of the junior level, the corresponding level objective would be: "Utilizes all steps of the nursing process in providing nursing care to individuals." When the educational program has three levels of nursing courses, a second level objective may be: "Utilizes the nursing process in providing nursing care for selected individuals." The implications for course objectives are obvious. Depending upon the faculty's orientation, the nursing courses in the program with three levels of nursing would have course objectives such as the following:

- Assesses the health status of the client in order to promote adaptation.
- Makes a nursing diagnosis based upon results of client assessment.
- Plans nursing care consistent with the nursing diagnosis, considering alternative nursing interventions.
- Promotes physiological adaptation by appropriate nursing intervention.
- Evaluates results of nursing intervention.

Obviously, these objectives are simple ones and are used here only to illustrate the curriculum process when nursing diagnosis has been identified as a step in the nursing process.

A legitimate question may well be: "Why nursing diagnosis instead of client problems?" "What is the value of a nursing diagnosis?" ask Durand and Prince (1966). Their answer is: "Nursing is seeking a scientific basis for practice. The process of diagnosing necessitates the use of scientific knowledge and requires the relation and application of this knowledge to nursing. The actual nursing diagnosis establishes a point of departure, a basis for nursing care."

Identification of client health problems is part of nursing diagnosis but nursing diagnosis encompasses more. It requires greater use of cognitive abilities because it requires the nurse to look beyond the immediate apparent health problem. For example, a client health problem may be: "Itching due to dry, flaking skin." The plan of care or nursing intervention may include a bath every five days and application of lotion to skin three times daily. A nursing diagnosis would take into account other variables such as the relationship of the client's dry skin to body image and effects of the client's response to his condition. Nursing diagnoses in this case might be:

1. Disturbance of body image caused by scaling skin.

2. Potential for skin impairment caused by scratching of skin.

Each of these diagnostic categories requires high degrees of assessment skills, knowledge of physiological functioning and psychological effect, and a variety of nursing interventions.

Nursing diagnosis involves a new way of thinking for nurses. It requires a systematized intellectual approach and implies an additional accountability for nursing actions because it reflects an independence of physician orders. It destines nurses to "think" as well as "do." According to Roy (1975), "Nursing diagnosis contributes to the nurse's quest for excellence by expanding knowledge, increasing sensitivity to human needs, allowing greater depth in self-understanding, emphasizing accountability to the consumer, and providing an overall awareness of issues affecting nursing and health care." It may appear that nursing diagnosis is the panacea for which nursing seeks. Although it cannot be that simple, Roy's point is well taken. It is the goal of nursing education to achieve that same excellence of which she speaks. On the other hand, Bircher (1975), in writing about the opponents of nursing diagnosis, states that these opponents fear premature diagnosis will result in "vagueness and inaccuracy" and "stereotyping," thus reducing individualized patient care. Bircher responds to the critics of diagnosis with the following: "In answer to the criticisms of diagnosis, it can be pointed out that the values or detriments of diagnosis are not inherent in diagnosis itself, but are functions of the cognitive adequacy or cognitive insufficiency of the user of the tool of diagnosis." Both Roy and Bircher imply the need for intellectual mastery of nursing knowledge, an uncontested goal of nursing education.

The implications for curriculum development are many if nursing diagnosis is a central component of the nursing process. The student must learn to integrate her knowledge of the physical, biological, and social sciences at an early stage in her educational preparation. "Even with a well delineated problem, such as potential skin breakdown, diagnosis requires the ability to consider multiple variables, each with different values, simultaneously" (Gordon, 1978). This necessitates fine implementation of a terminal objective frequently stated in nursing programs: engages in critical thinking in arriving at a course of nursing action. Nursing diagnosis requires critical thinking as well as high levels of conceptualization. Diagnosis becomes the end product of assessment and helps the nurse to describe the health state of the client. Gordon (1976) states: "Many nurses tend to talk about a patient's health problem in terms of functional concepts like 'needs assurance' or 'provide adequate oxygenation,' rather than to specify the problem first. One way to shift emphasis is to ask why this person needs reassurance, suctioning, or any other nursing activity. The answer is a description of the client state — anticipatory anxiety or potential respiratory obstruction." Certainly, the goal of describing the client state is not new to nursing, and it is the foundation upon which nursing diagnosis is built.

The next steps of the nursing process, *planning*, *intervention*, and *evaluation*, are dependent upon the nursing diagnosis. The diagnosis gives direction for planning, and the intervention is based upon it. Given an accurate nursing diagnosis, the evaluation step of the nursing process is an uncomplicated one. If the evaluation reveals that signs and symptoms have diminished or have been eliminated, nursing intervention has been effective.

Inclusion of the concept of nursing diagnosis into a curriculum provides opportunities for students to meet level or terminal objectives other than those directly related to this concept. Communication among colleagues and other health care providers is consistently a goal of nursing education. *Nursing diagnosis requires collaboration among nurses.* They must learn to confer with each other in order to corroborate their diagnoses and the signs and symptoms that precipitated the labeling. For example, a statement of a level objective might be: "collaborates with peers." Nursing diagnosis provides a vehicle for this by requiring students to problem-solve with each other by sharing information about various alterations they observe and fitting these into diagnostic categories. The locus of information-sharing becomes one of collaboration rather than simply of communication.

A second typical objective of nursing diagnosis regards the accountability of nurses. Nursing students must be held accountable for their actions as students, and they must be prepared to assume accountability as professionals. Nursing diagnosis provides a unique opportunity because it requires the nurse to hold her actions up for scrutiny by others as well as to share her knowledge while seeking more information. Like collaboration, accountability requires the nurse, student, or professional practitioner to engage in scientific problem-solving, which implies logical thinking and exacting decision-making.

Another objective that has become more universal within the past few years concerns the nurse's understanding of the research process. Regardless of the expected degrees of sophisticated research behaviors of the nursing student, nursing diagnosis has major implications. If an expected terminal behavior is the demonstration of ability to participate in the research process, the student can help collect data regarding the relationship between a particular diagnosis and its signs and symptoms. Should an expected terminal behavior be one of conducting research, the student has an opportunity to engage in experimental research that may show a relationship between nursing interventions and client outcomes.

One of the primary prerequisites for inclusion of nursing diagnosis in the curriculum is the faculty's knowledge of and skill in the nursing diagnostic process. Students must have as role models faculty who can keenly discern between conceptualizing and theorizing, between intuitive knowledge and scientific methodology. If nursing diagnosis requires, as the literature states, a new way of thinking for nurses, the faculty who are preparing tomorrow's practitioners must be able to engage in high levels of intellectualization, as well as exercise exceptionally refined judgment. In addition, they must be expert in all components of the nursing process and in their own practice of nursing.

Finally, *nursing diagnosis presents an opportunity for nursing to be recognized as an autonomous profession because diagnosis represents autonomy of nursing practice.* No longer relying solely upon the medical diagnosis for determining nursing intervention, nurses will assume responsibility not only for keen assessment of an observable condition but also for hypothesizing the causes of that condition. Once diagnostic categories are established, nurses can institute nursing intervention in an independent manner.

The incorporation of nursing diagnosis into a curriculum requires all the intellectual skills of making a nursing diagnosis in addition to a knowledge of curriculum development and the teaching-learning process. It is no small task and requires a philosophical commitment on the part of the nursing faculty who will be implementing the curriculum.

References:

Aspinall, M.J.: Nursing diagnosis — The weak link. *Nursing Outlook, 24*:433, 1976.

Bircher, A.U.: On the development and classification of diagnoses. *Nursing Forum, 14*:10, 1975.

Durand, M., and Prince, R.: Nursing diagnosis: Process and decision. *Nursing Forum, 5*:58, 1966.

Gordon, M.: Classification of nursing diagnoses. *Journal, N.Y. State Nurses' Association, 9*:5, 1978.

Gordon, M.: Nursing diagnosis and the diagnostic process. *Am. J. Nurs.*, 1298, 1976.

Roy, C.: The impact of nursing diagnosis. *AORN Journal, 21*:1023, 1975.

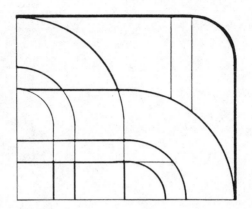

SECTION THREE

NURSING DIAGNOSIS:

Client Models for
Utilization

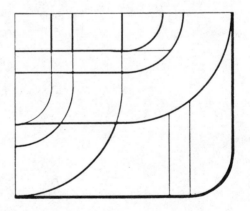

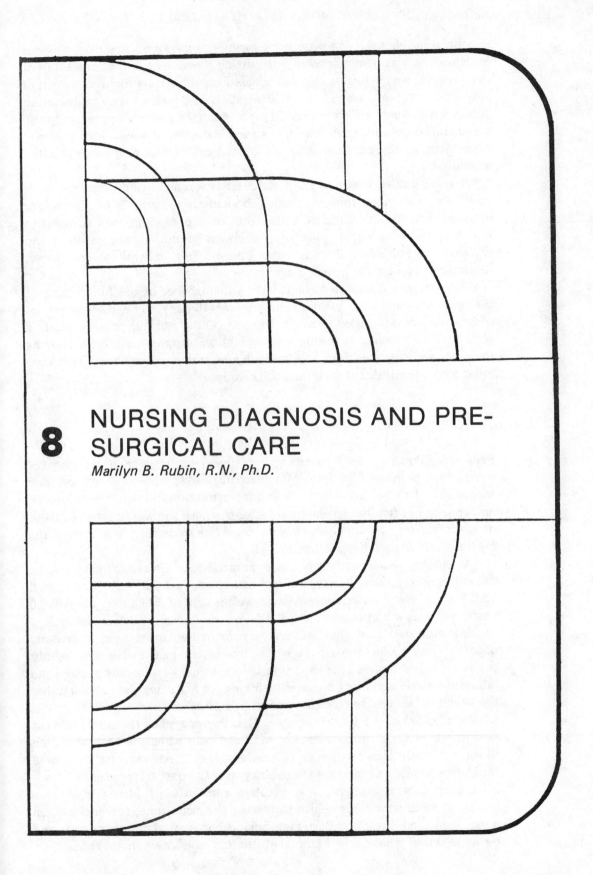

8 NURSING DIAGNOSIS AND PRE-SURGICAL CARE

Marilyn B. Rubin, R.N., Ph.D.

In a previous chapter, the process of formulation of a nursing diagnosis was explained. It was demonstrated that nursing assessment is the initial step of this process, which in this chapter is based on the conceptual framework of adaptation of man. Assessment of adaptation of the client is an examination of the individual's ability to modify physiological, psychological, cultural, social, and developmental behaviors to meet the requirements for successful adjustment to the environment, life events, or internal changes within the individual.

It is concluded that a healthy state exists when this individual responds positively to changes while continuing to maintain integrity in all dimensions of adaptation. In an individual's life, from day to day and even moment to moment, there is continuous adaptation to stimuli in the internal and external environment. Through the optimal use of available resources, maximum potential for health is achieved.

This chapter discusses a client with a disturbance of the functioning of the gall bladder that resulted in surgical therapy. The dimensions of adaptation are identified through the use of the nursing process, starting with assessment and concluding with evaluation or outcome criteria. Nursing therapies are suggested for the admission and pre-operative phases. Outcome criteria are identified for each nursing therapy.

CLIENT SITUATION

Frequently, malfunctions of the gall bladder result in an acute stage of discomfort, pain, and anxiety. Mrs. Barbara Porter was no exception. She was admitted to the hospital on a Sunday afternoon following an enjoyable dinner with her family. Several hours after the meal she was in acute distress, necessitating care in the emergency room. After examining Mrs. Porter, the medical staff advised hospitalization.

A nursing assessment was made immediately after admission to the patient care unit. Mrs. Porter, a blond caucasian, was 5'5" tall. She weighed 72.7 kg, which she stated represented a weight gain of 20 kg over the past 15 years. She is now 35 years old and a wife and mother in a nuclear family.

She indicated that she had severe pain in her upper right abdominal quadrant just below the rib cage and less severe pain in the area of her posterior left shoulder (Fig. 8–1). In the emergency room, she received an intramuscular injection of meperidine 50 mg for her pain. She indicated that the injection had relieved her discomfort to a great extent.

When asked about food tolerance, Mrs. Porter replied that she could eat most foods but had noticed similar, localized pain when she had eaten rich foods, especially those with high fat content. Mrs. Porter reported that these food intolerances had increased in severity over the past six months.

During this assessment, the adaptive responses of Mrs. Porter were examined to ascertain her health status. At the same time, the professional nurse identified that Mrs. Porter seemed capable of dynamic change and recognized that what seemed factual at the first assessment might change.

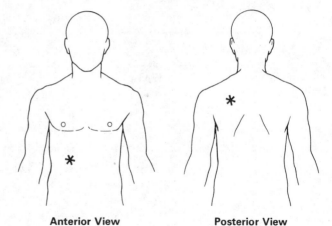

Figure 8-1 Identified areas of abdominal and shoulder pain.

Anterior View   Posterior View

In assessing the adaptive responses of Mrs. Porter, the following questions were considered:

- Are the individual's responses adequate?
- Are the individual's responses deficient?
- Are the individual's responses excessive?
- Are the individual's responses inappropriate?
- Are there dysfunctional factors that prevent or distort response?

The descriptive words adequate, deficient, excessive, inappropriate and dysfunctional indicate the level to which Mrs. Porter is currently able to adapt to her altered health state.

An *adequate* response indicates that Mrs. Porter has been able to meet necessary requirements through her own resources to maintain herself when stimulated by external or internal changes.

If Mrs. Porter were unable to maintain herself without resources provided by other persons, then she would be in a state that may be assessed as *deficient*. An *excessive* response indicates that the individual has gone beyond normal limits of a behavior in any of the dimensions of adaptation. *Inappropriate* responses indicate that the individual does not or cannot respond in a manner that solves the problem of adaptation. *Dysfunctional* factors are those that the individual has no way to respond to; for example, an amputated leg produces a situation in which the individual is immobile unless provided resources such as crutches, prosthesis, or a wheelchair. A *distorted* response occurs when normal function is inhibited by sensory misinterpretation, anatomical deformity, or disfigurement. In a social sense, the individual's roles in life may be disorganized.

The dimensions of adaptation used for major categories of assessment for Mrs. Porter are indicated in Table 8–1.

Following admission, Mrs. Porter had diagnostic tests, including x-rays of the gall bladder that confirmed the presence of gallstones. It was noted that the gall bladder had demonstrated a delayed delivery of bile, when needed,

Table 8–1 Assessment Categories: Dimensions of Adaptation

Dimensions	Behaviors
Physiological	Physiological systems exist to regulate functions to maintain life. Behaviors include a range of dynamic physiological adaptations to respond to or modify stimuli from internal or external environments.
Psychological	Appropriate interpersonal and self-regulating behaviors maintain the unity and integrity of the individual so that life can be experienced fully. Spiritual characteristics reflect the individual's belief system consisting of religious, ethical, and moral values that are useful to the individual in adapting to living in the contemporary world.
Cultural	The cultural dimension exemplifies the traditional heritage of the individual, reflected in various ethnic behaviors.
Social	The social aspects of the individual include behaviors that are appropriate for effective relationships with individuals and groups within the community. These people may be helpful resources for the individual in need of adaptation.
Developmental	These behaviors indicate the individual's level of development. Adaptation from birth to old age requires changes in behavior, that is, developmental tasks that are dynamic and appropriate to the individual and the specific stage of development.

to the intestine. No outstanding deviations were noted in the blood and urine studies.

The major alteration of adaptation identified for Mrs. Porter was that her gall bladder was not functioning adequately. This was probably caused by the presence of the stones in the gall bladder, which impeded the normal flow of bile necessary for effective fat digestion.

In talking with Mrs. Porter, she revealed that she was anxious about the impending surgery (cholecystectomy), which was to take place on the following day. Her anxiety stemmed from her concern about her ability to function after recovery and whether or not cancer would be discovered. Dr. Mary Hart, her physician, told her that she did not anticipate the presence of cancer.

When asked about the ease with which she could rest in the hospital, Mrs. Porter said that she enjoyed reading to pass the time when she did not have visitors. She was frequently disturbed from her sleep at night by the nurse giving care to the patient in the adjacent bed. Her sleep was further hampered by extraneous noise from personnel and their activities because her room was located near the nurses' desk. She slept for short periods in the late afternoon when she became tired.

Dimensions of Adaptation

Adaptive Responses	Physiological	Psychological	Cultural	Developmental	Social
Adequate			X	X	X
Deficient	X	X			
Excessive		X			
Inappropriate		X			
Dysfunctional	X				

3 2 1	3 2 1	③② 1	③②①	③ 2 ①

Level of Adaptive Resources

Figure 8–2 Nursing Assessment of Mrs. Porter Using Adaptation Dimensions.
3 = Individual; *2* = Family; *1* = Community.

Mrs. Porter indicated that she felt guilty in not having attended to her spiritual concerns for some time. She was baptized in the Catholic Church and confirmed in the Lutheran Church. She now attended the Baptist Church on an irregular basis. She requested to see a Lutheran clergyman before going to surgery.

While collecting data from Mrs. Porter, the professional nurse used an assessment data sheet (Fig. 8-2). Each of the dimensions of adaptation is examined along the scale of adaptive responses.

NURSING ASSESSMENT DATA BASE

The significant conclusions drawn from Mrs. Porter's assessment data base are discussed in the following paragraphs.

Physiological Dimension of Adaptation

Adaptive Response

Deficient   Mrs. Porter experienced pain from contraction of the gall bladder as a result of irritation from stones.

Mrs. Porter experienced a disturbed sleep cycle. Her usual circadian rhythm of night sleep was interrupted by noise in and outside of her hospital room.

Dysfunctional — The digestive function of the gastrointestinal tract was disturbed, particularly fat digestion.

Mrs. Porter was unable to tolerate fat ingestion in her diet at this time. Lipid metabolism was impaired because fat was not digested properly.

Psychological Dimension of Adaptation

Adaptive Response

Deficient — Mrs. Porter demonstrated restless motions of hands and frequent shifting in posture.

Mrs. Porter's illness made her think of her spiritual life, and she expressed guilt feelings about neglecting this aspect of her life.

Excessive — Mrs. Porter's hands were cold to touch, and she perspired excessively.

Mrs. Porter's eyes frequently shifted in gaze as she looked about the room.

Inappropriate — Mrs. Porter continued to eat rich foods, even though her physician recommended avoiding fatty foods in her diet.

Cultural Dimension of Adaptation

Adaptive Response

Adequate — Mrs. Porter was of German heritage. She stated that she was "content" with her role in her family. Mrs. Porter enjoyed cooking German food for her family.

Developmental Dimension of Adaptation

Adaptive Response

Adequate — Mrs. Porter stated that she enjoyed being a wife and mother. She was satisfied with the tasks of the homemaker and had no desire for a career outside the home.

She indicated that functions within the nuclear family assisted her in generativity.

Social Dimension of Adaptation

Adaptive Response

Adequate   Mrs. Porter expressed satisfaction with relationships with friends. She was secretary of the Parent-Teachers Association at the school that her children attended.

By examining Figure 8–2, it is clearly seen that the major health care problems of Mrs. Porter are deficiencies in the adaptive responses for the physiological and psychological dimensions of adaptation. There is also a dysfunctional adaptive response in the physiological dimension and excessive and inappropriate adaptive responses in the psychological dimension. In the positive realm, Mrs. Porter indicated an adequate adaptive response in the cultural, developmental, and social dimensions of adaptation.

NURSING DIAGNOSIS

The first step of the nursing process, assessment, is necessary to determine the nursing diagnoses for Mrs. Porter. According to the listing of nursing diagnoses by the National Group for Classification of Nursing Diagnosis (1977) and the data collected, the following *nursing diagnoses* are given:

1. Anxiety
2. Coping, ineffective
3. Guilt, related to religious beliefs
4. Nutritional alterations
5. Pain
6. Changes in sleep-rest cycle

When formulating nursing diagnoses, it is important to remember that this event is not a one-time phenomenon but rather a dynamic process. Nursing diagnoses change as they reflect the dynamic state of the individual and the progression of adaptive abilities.

NURSING PLAN, INTERVENTION, EVALUATION

As the professional nurse proceeds with nursing process, the next steps include the planning and implementing of nursing therapy and evaluation of the client responses according to outcome criteria.

In the planning phase, the professional nurse reviews the assessment data and nursing diagnosis. She uses these as a basis for planning care. Resources of self, family, and community that the client is using for adaptation are recognized, and other resources are sought for areas in which adaptive responses are deficient, inappropriate, excessive, or dysfunctional.

Nursing interventions for Mrs. Porter are based upon the previously cited nursing diagnoses. Nursing therapy is categorized in four areas in the conceptual framework of adaptation. Goals used for planning nursing intervention in relation to adaptation include:

- Promotion of adaptation
- Correction and/or assistance for correction of inadequate responses
- Support of appropriate responses
- Provision of resources

In relation to the physiological dimension, the nursing diagnoses of pain, changes in sleep-wake cycle, and nutritional alterations reflected both dysfunction and deficiency. Mrs. Porter has pain (deficiency), the circadian rhythm of the sleep-rest cycle is disturbed (deficiency), and her digestive function and lipid metabolism are maladaptive (dysfunctional).

The *goals* for nursing therapy previously listed are examined, and those considered to be priorities are selected. The nurse chooses the following goals: (1) to promote adaptation to pain, (2) to support an adaptive response to the circadian rhythm sleep-rest cycle, and (3) to assist in the correction of dysfunctional digestive responses.

Mrs. Porter's response of pain to the dysfunctional gall bladder indicates that her body alerted her to inherent physiological changes. Although Mrs. Porter's pain was relieved temporarily through analgesics, permanent relief of pain had to be achieved through excision of the dysfunctional tissues and removal of gall stones. Other supportive nursing therapy includes discussing the pain experience, decreasing the anxiety level, providing comfort measures to increase well-being, and supporting the sleep cycle.

Mrs. Porter may choose to move to another room where she may be either alone in the room or with a roommate who is less disturbing. Maintaining and supporting Mrs. Porter's pre-sleep rituals such as teeth brushing, other personal hygiene activities, reading before sleep, and providing uninterrupted sleep according to her pre-hospital sleep cycle are nursing therapies not to be overlooked. Decreasing the noise in the ambient environment to less than 45 decibels provides a positive factor for the sleep cycle (Acre and Rubin, 1977).

Dysfunctional digestion resulted from a disturbed gall bladder and the presence of gall stones. The professional nurse provided supports to Mrs. Porter's adaptive responses by serving a prescribed low-fat diet and by supporting the physician and nutritionist in teaching Mrs. Porter about her dietary requirements, pre- and postoperatively.

Mrs. Porter previously ignored her own individual resources to delete fatty, rich foods from her diet. Other resources that she now uses are those of the physician, nutritionist, and nurse to reach this goal. The *outcome criteria* of the previously stated nursing therapies included:

- Temporary relief of pain
- Restoration of the sleep cycle
- Tolerance of low-fat diet

In the psychological dimension of adaptation, deficient, excessive, and inappropriate adaptive responses were identified that supported the nursing diagnoses of *anxiety*, *ineffective coping behaviors*, and *guilt related to religious beliefs*.

The nursing therapy provided by the professional nurse explored and assisted Mrs. Porter in identifying and explaining the anxiety behavior. Together they discussed the cause of her anxiety. She already identified impending surgery and the possiblity of the diagnosis of carcinoma as major causes.

The professional nurse supported her coping behavior of reading as a means of decreasing the anxiety. The professional nurse may also employ other resources such as the family or community to assist Mrs. Porter to modify her behavior.

Mrs. Porter herself is considered a resource when she is drawn into discussion about previous activities that she used to relieve anxiety. The professional nurse encouraged Mrs. Porter to formulate a pattern for coping in this situation that included herself, her family and the community. She already indicated that she sought the resource of Dr. Hart, who said that there was no evidence of carcinoma.

Mrs. Porter expressed her feelings of guilt in not having maintained a spiritual relationship between God and herself. The feelings of guilt were supported and amplified by thoughts of her illness, suffering, and impending surgery.

The nursing care plan included activities that were designed to assist Mrs. Porter in meeting her spiritual needs, and this allowed her to experience a closer alliance with God.

The professional nurse explored the spiritual aspects with Mrs. Porter to assist her to identify the causes for her guilt and to assist in a plan to resolve Mrs. Porter's feelings of guilt. The professional nurse also assisted Mrs. Porter by supporting her spirituality through prayer and meditative reading. Uninterrupted time was provided for the support of Mrs. Porter through family devotion and religious discussion. Community resources were utilized when Mrs. Porter requested the minister of her choice.

The desired *outcome criteria* for these nursing therapies included:

- Relaxed postural musculature
- Relaxed facial expression
- Warm, moderately moist hands
- Normal heart rate
- Normal blood pressure
- Normal respiratory rate and rhythm
- Meditation on religious materials

- Reactivated religious practice, that is, celebration of religious sacraments, prayer, attendance at religious service
- Verbal expressions of hope

In the cultural, developmental, and social dimensions of adaptation, Mrs. Porter was assessed as adequate. Therefore, the professional nurse continued to promote Mrs. Porter's activities to maintain adaptation in these areas. Obviously, her community activities were discontinued during her hospitalization. Her roles as wife and mother continued throughout the hospitalization. The nurse supported these roles by encouraging visits and psychological support by the family.

Since Mrs. Porter had the benefit of the previously mentioned nursing therapies and demonstrated the desired outcomes, she went to surgery for a cholecystectomy in an adaptive state. Her adaptive responses were enhanced by the nurse's assistance in correcting inadequate responses, supporting appropriate responses, and providing resources when Mrs. Porter could not.

SUMMARY

In this chapter, it was demonstrated that nursing diagnoses have a significant function in clarifying and directing nursing therapies to be used for an individual in the pre-operative phase prior to cholecystectomy. Nursing diagnoses were used as an integral part of the nursing process, and this process was used within the organizational constructs of the conceptual framework of adaptation of man.

References:

Acre, E.M., and Rubin, M.: Sleep disturbance from environmental noise. *Transactions of the Illinois State Academy of Science,* 70:213, 1977.

Rubin, M.: *Nursing Care for Myocardial Infarction.* St. Louis, Warren H. Green, Inc., 1977.

Way, L.: Diseases of the gallbladder and bile ducts. *In* Beeson, McDermott, and Wyngaarden (eds.): *Cecil Textbook of Medicine.* Philadelphia, W.B. Saunders, Co., 1979.

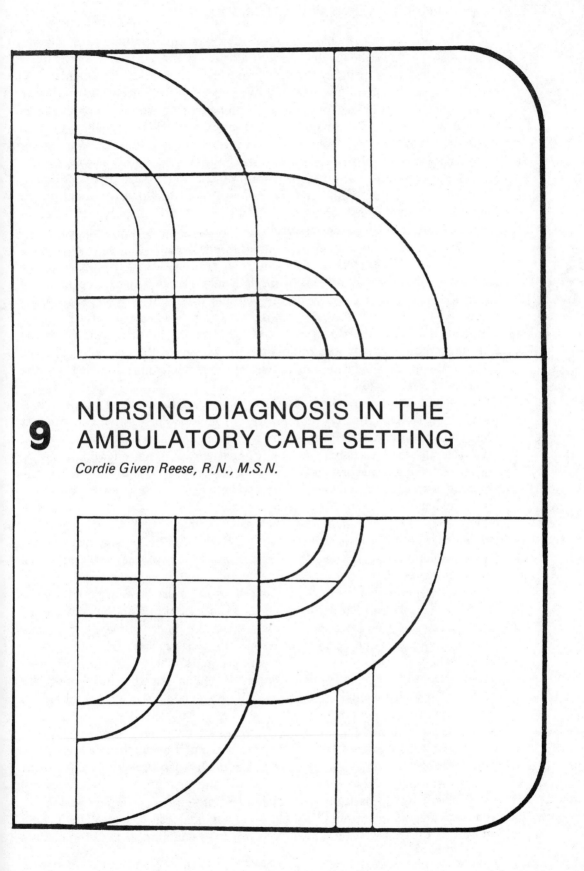

9 NURSING DIAGNOSIS IN THE AMBULATORY CARE SETTING

Cordie Given Reese, R.N., M.S.N.

The purpose of this chapter is to illustrate the usefulness of nursing diagnosis by the independent nurse practitioner. This author views the nurse practitioner as a primary health provider for a group of clients with predominantly nursing needs. The nurse may consult with other health care personnel but practices nursing in an independent manner. For example, consultations may be made with the physician when a client's medical condition deteriorates, with a social worker about community resources, or with a dietitian if the client demonstrates complicated dietary needs.

Inherent in the term primary care provider is the concept of continuity of care and working with the client for an extended period of time. Primary care also addresses the concept of health promotion, health maintenance, and alleviation of those factors that cause illness (Robischon, 1966).

The setting in which the nurse practitioner works, often in an outpatient facility, forces the nurse to view the client from different perspectives. The client is often not as passive in other health care settings as he is in the hospital and is more free to decide whether to accept or reject the nurse's services. As a result, involving the client in decisions about health care is crucial. Since the decisions are made with the nurse, the client views the nurse as more directly accountable for the success of the plan of care. Thus, the nurse must anticipate and answer the client's inquiries concerning the failure of intervention.

Since making a nursing diagnosis is part of the nursing process, it is important to recognize the framework in which this process will be used. As previously noted, a conceptual framework of adaptation is used in this book. By identifying the changes in the internal and external environment that affect the client (assessment) and labeling them (nursing diagnosis), the practitioner acts to enhance the ability of the client to adapt by planning, intervening, and evaluating nursing therapies. If the client later arrives at a high adaptive level using the resources available, that is, if the client demonstrates an improved health status, both from his perspective and the practitioner's point of view, the client is more adaptive than before, and the practitioner evaluates the process as being successful.

To give effective care, the nursing diagnosis must be considered openly and consciously to plan and provide interventions based on the synthesis of information derived from the assessment data. In reality, nurses *always* make a diagnosis, for one cannot intervene without having first come to a conclusion. However, often these conclusions are not conscious or well-conceptualized. The nursing diagnosis is crucial to the success of the functioning of the nurse practitioner. If the nursing diagnosis is incorrect, interventions will seldom succeed.

The steps in making a nursing diagnosis are many and complex and may vary with the cognitive style of the assessor. First, as much data as possible are gathered and analyzed; judgments are made about selection of pertinent assessment data, which are then grouped and examined for relationships, critical attributes, patterns, and organizing principles. After comparing the chosen category to normative data, a nursing diagnosis is made. The nursing diagnosis then becomes the focal point for the remaining steps of the nursing process.

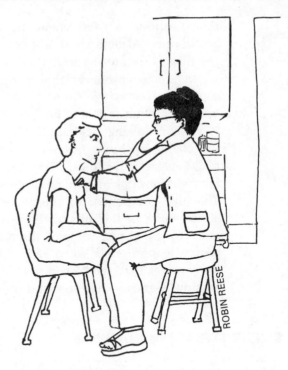

ROBIN REESE

This chapter utilizes the following processes to conceptualize and formulate a nursing diagnosis. First, a short concluding statement of the synthesis of assessment data is presented. When appropriate, previously published nursing diagnosis nomenclature is used. Second, the nursing diagnosis is given an etiology. Third, the appropriate signs and symptoms are described. This process of formulating diagnoses has proven satisfactory for both health maintenance and illness diagnoses.

Since health is no longer considered as only the absence of biological disease, it is important to evaluate and support healthy states as well as conquer illness. Literature reflects little emphasis on healthy states as compared to the vast amount of information available concerning disease. Wellness-illness can be perceived as a continuum, with a step-wise progression from health or wellness to illness. Dunn (1959) describes these steps: (1) the optimally healthy person, (2) the healthy person in an unhealthy environment, (3) an ill person in a healthy environment or a protected person, and (4) an ill person in an unhealthy environment. Berg (1979) discusses the same continuum but describes healthy and unhealthy diagnoses along this continuum.

Another way to view health is to identify the client's positive health factors. These factors are those assessment parameters within the individual that are healthy. Assessing both healthy and unhealthy parameters in the same person gives the practitioner a total view of the client and allows for the formulation of diagnoses useful for the maintenance and promotion of health. Nursing diagnoses for health maintenance are used as conclusions derived from healthy factors identified in the history and examination. Interventions for these diagnoses and related goals center around supporting those actions of the client that promote health and discussing other health-oriented actions of which the client may not be aware. Examples of the diagnostic process in illness and health are (1) alterations in circulation secondary to coronary atherosclerosis manifested by chest pain and (2) a supportive family system secondary to a family who cares, demonstrated by open communication and family members assisting one another.

The following case studies demonstrate nursing diagnoses appropriate for clients with cardiovascular disease; they are related to both health maintenance and illness. The case studies are designed to demonstrate the interrelationships of nursing diagnosis to other steps of the nursing process. The final component of the nursing process, evaluation, helps validate the effectiveness of the nursing diagnosis and thus fosters accountability by the nurse to the client. Some of the nursing diagnoses presented in this chapter proved inappropriate when evaluation occurred; in these instances, the data were reorganized and analyzed in an effort to formulate more accurate nursing diagnoses and successful results.

CLIENT SITUATION: Mrs. White

Mrs. White ia a 71 year old patient with a history of alcoholism, asthma, myocardial infarction, and pancreatitis. She lives alone. The client sees herself as ill and in need of help, and she views the nurse as one who can help. Her family is important to her, but she feels they neither like her nor are supportive of her. Comments: "I am alone; my family doesn't care. I have no friends. Why shouldn't I drink? It helps the pains." Upon clarification, "pains" referred to physical aches and the suffering of feeling lonely. She smokes one-half pack of cigarettes a day and admits to wheezing, dyspnea, and the production of a small amount of clear sputum nearly every morning since childhood. She states that these attacks increase with emotional activity and are relieved with ephedrine. She denies chest and abdominal pain and any changes in orthopnea or nocturia. She says she has been drinking approximately a fifth of whiskey a day for one year.

Assessment

The physical examination reveals a woman of small stature with a staggering gait, slurred speech, accurate orientation, and a sad expression. She has a normal temperature, a regular heart rate of 100/minute, a blood pressure of 130/70, no jugular venous distention (JVD) while in an upright position, normal heart sounds, no pedal edema, and an abdominal exam within normal limits. She does have expiratory musical rales (crackles) and slightly decreased air exchange.

Laboratory data reveal a normal SMA 12, normal blood electrolytes, and a normal CBC. A chest x-ray was normal. The electrocardiogram shows Q waves in leads II, III, and AVF. The amylase level is normal at 70 Somogyi units.

Three nursing diagnoses were derived from the assessment data:

1. Loneliness secondary to perceptions of having no support systems, manifested by feelings of being alone and unhappy.

2. Hypoxia secondary to decreased ventilation, manifested by rales (crackles) and a decrease in air exchange.

3. Maintenance of independence secondary to viewing herself as self-sufficient, manifested by living alone for many years.

NURSING DIAGNOSIS

Loneliness secondary to perceptions of having no support stytem, manifested by feelings of being alone and unhappy.

Plan

For the nursing diagnosis of loneliness, the plan is to increase Mrs. White's interaction with other people, thereby decreasing her feelings of loneliness, increasing her feelings of self-worth, and decreasing the anxiety that is initiated by the loneliness and dissipated by drinking.

Intervention

Nursing Interventions	Outcome Criteria
1. Uses self as a support system to client by being available anytime by telephone and seeing the client 2 to 3 times per week.	1. Client will telephone the nurse for support and will stop drinking in six months.
2. Encourage other forms of interaction such as talking with family, friends, and persons from church and neighborhood center.	2. Client will increase interactions by developing one more friendship, attending one club regularly during a three month period, and by verbalizing one or two positive feelings about self at each visit with the nurse.

Evaluation

The evaluation revealed that Mrs. White stopped drinking regularly after two months and had only an occasional beer after one year. She sees her family from time to time, makes one or two positive statements about herself regularly, and goes to church at least once a month with a friend.

_____ NURSING DIAGNOSIS _____

Hypoxia secondary to decreased ventilation, manifested by rales (crackles) and a decrease in air exchange.

Plan

For the nursing diagnosis, hypoxia, the plan is to decrease airway resistance and increase oxygen exchange.

Intervention

Nursing Interventions	*Outcome Criteria*
1. Give information concerning the use, action, and hazards of ephedrine.	1. Client will take fewer than fifteen ephedrine a month and will describe the appropriate use of ephedrine.
2. Tell client that the nurse is available by telephone, thereby decreasing the patient's anxiety and respiratory distress caused by feeling alone.	2. Client will call the nurse at least once between office visits, and the number of asthmatic attacks will decrease after the nurse-client interaction is initiated.
3. Discuss the need to increase fluid intake to liquefy pulmonary secretions and decrease airway resistance.	3. Client will report drinking 2000 cc of fluid per day.
4. Teach client to monitor ankles to assess for overhydration.	4. Client will verbalize knowledge gained from the patient teaching; nurse and client will assess ankles together at each office visit.
5. Teach hazards of catching colds and of smoking, which increase airway resistance and decrease oxygen exchange.	5. Client will have fewer colds over the next six months compared to last year and will lessen the number of cigarettes smoked by decreasing them at the rate of one cigarette a day, starting one month from initial visit.
6. Teach breathing exercises to increase aeration in the lungs.	6. Client will return the demonstration at every office visit.

Evaluation

The evaluation of this nursing diagnosis showed that Mrs. White's airway resistance decreased, which was manifested in the following ways: her expiratory wheezes disappeared; she took fewer than fifteen ephedrine a month; she used the emergency room less than she did a year ago to treat her asthmatic attacks. She also had fewer colds than she had over the same time period a year ago. She is able to assess her ankles accurately for pedal edema, and she reports drinking ten large glasses of fluid a day. Mrs. White has not decreased her smoking, nor can she completely return the breathing exercise demonstration. She states that this is because she does not see the importance of these interventions.

_____ **NURSING DIAGNOSIS** _____

Maintenance of independence secondary to viewing herself as self-sufficient, manifested by living alone for many years.

Plan

For the nursing diagnosis of maintenance of independence, the plan is to reinforce and support this independence.

Intervention

Nursing Interventions	*Outcome Criteria*
1. Praise her past abilities and present efforts to remain independent.	1. Client will demonstrate pleasure by smiling and agreeing with nurse.
2. Manipulate present environment to allow client to continue living alone by providing transportation, easy access to health care, someone with whom to discuss problems, opportunities for recreation, and less costly grocery services.	2. Client will regularly make use of transportation, health care, support person, and recreation and other services within two months.
3. Allow client to assist in her health care planning, thereby encouraging her self-sufficiency.	3. Client will collaborate with the nurse in determining details for care plan starting with the first office visit.

Evaluation

Evaluation of Mrs. White's situation finds her living at home, and she is satisfied with her decision. She uses the services provided and offers input into her care at every office visit.

Review of three nursing diagnoses shows that they are accurate. The nursing care evaluations demonstrated that the interventions derived from the nursing diagnoses were successful.

CLIENT SITUATION: Mr. Smith

Mr. Smith is a 5'4", 50 year old client who weighs 320 pounds. His medical diagnoses are angina, hypertension, cardiomyopathy, and history of heavy alcohol intake.

In relating his symptoms, Mr. Smith states that he feels he is retaining fluid and that he urinates less. He sleeps on three pillows, a change from his previous use of two pillows last week, and he experiences paroxysmal nocturnal dyspnea. He notes no chest pain and denies any intake of alcohol. He states that he has difficulty obtaining an erection, which he attributes to the diuretic. Periodically he expresses the concern that his wife will be upset with their inability to have intercourse easily and regularly. He does take his other medications, methyldopa and hydralazine. Client does not read or write. A verbal diet history reveals that he had a high caloric intake, high sodium meals, and snacks the previous day. He explains that he enjoys food, especially with his friends, that his wife is obese and likes to cook, and that his children eat fruits and vegetables bought for him. He states that he knows the relationship between calories and weight, but he demonstrates little knowledge of the relationship between number of calories, salt in specific foods, and serving size. The following information was gleaned during a previous home visit: use of foods very high in carbohydrates and high in sodium content, little understanding of illness by client's family, low income, and children in home who eat up all fresh fruits and vegetables.

On this examination, the nurse finds no change in speech, sensation, motor, or behavior patterns that might indicate a CVA. His face is not edematous; JVD is 4 cm above the clavicle when the client is in an upright position; H.R. is 100 with 6 to 7 premature beats per minute. He has fine inspiratory rales (crackles) heard one quarter of the way up the back, which do not change with coughing. His liver is enlarged and his girth has increased by seven inches. The right foot demonstrates 3+ edema up to the mid-calf. The left foot provides unreliable data because of a venous ulcer. B.P. is 150/85, and S_3 is noted. In one week his weight has increased 13 pounds.

Laboratory tests demonstrate normal SGPT, SGOT, and CPK. Serum sodium is 128 mEq/L; potassium is 3.0 mEq/L; and digoxin level is 1.9 mg/ml. Chest x-ray reveals scattered densities indicative of congestive heart failure. Electrocardiogram shows sinus tachycardia with 6 to 8 premature atrial beats per minute.

The nursing diagnoses for Mr. Smith are:

1. Alterations in cardiac output secondary to cardiomyopathy, manifested by orthopnea, paroxysmal nocturnal dyspnea, pedal edema, increased girth, S_3, tachycardia, rales (crackles), enlarged liver, and increased JVD.

2. Impotence secondary to drug intake, manifested by slow attainment of erection.

NURSING DIAGNOSIS

Alterations in cardiac output secondary to cardiomyopathy, manifested by orthopnea, paroxysmal nocturnal dyspnea, pedal edema, increased girth, S_3, tachycardia, rales (crackles), enlarged liver, and increased JVD.

Plan

For the nursing diagnosis of alterations in cardiac output, the plan is to increase oxygen available to the myocardium by decreasing body requirements for oxygen.

Intervention

Nursing Interventions	Outcome Criteria
1. Identify client's values regarding food with high calories and sodium content.	1. Client will list food preferences, taste preferences, and cooking techniques at first visit.
2. Instruct client to record 24-hour diet history.	2. At every visit, client will bring diet history.
3. Outline activity schedule allowing for long rest periods.	3. Client will discuss schedule that fits his life style and will review it with practitioner.
4. Clarify values regarding alcohol intake and describe its effect on the heart.	4. Client will discuss feelings about, needs for, situations leading to drinking. He will verbalize its effects on his heart.
5. Discuss need, action, and side effects of diuretic, digoxin, and potassium.	5. Client will lose 5 to 10 pounds in one week. Digoxin level will remain less than 2 mg. Potassium will remain at 3.5 to 5 mEq/L.
6. Discuss with client at every visit the need to take drugs as ordered.	6. Heart rhythm will be normal sinus, with no more than five atrial premature beats per minute.
7. Instruct client in 1500 calorie low-sodium diet.	7. Client will lose 1 to 2 pounds per week indefinitely and will verbalize a 24-hour diet recall of no use of sodium products every week.

Evaluation

Evaluation revealed disappearance of the S_3, rales (crackles), and tachycardia, indicating that there was increased oxygen available to the myocardium. In addition, the client's girth and peripheral edema decreased. A steady weight loss was not attained, even though eight pounds were lost the first week.

_____ NURSING DIAGNOSIS _____

Impotence secondary to drug intake, manifested by slow attainment of erection.

Plan

For the nursing diagnosis of impotence, the plan is to increase sexual satisfaction, thereby increasing the quality of life.

Intervention

Nursing Interventions	Outcome Criteria
1. Discuss need for the maintenance of diuretic therapy, because an increase in fluid retention increases the load on the heart.	1. Client will not gain more than 1 to 2 pounds of weight by the next week, and peripheral edema will not be evidenced.
2. Nurse will consult with physician about reducing dosage of methyldopa, which has a side effect of decreased libido.	2. Client will verbalize an increase in ability to have and maintain an erection. Client will not have B.P. greater than 140/90.
3. Give patient permission to discuss feelings regarding this matter with the practitioner and encourage him to discuss his feelings with his wife.	3. Client will discuss feelings and verbalize an increase in sexual satisfaction.

Evaluation

Evaluation demonstrates that the patient did verbalize an increase in sexual satisfaction, and according to his weight, maintained his diuretic therapy. In examining the failure of Mr. Smith to lose weight consistently, the practitioner had to re-evaluate her nursing diagnosis. By reviewing the assessment data, the nurse assumed that Mr. Smith's statement of desire to lose weight would evolve into the appropriate behavior. Since this did not occur, an evaluation of the nursing process must occur. In this case, an additional nursing diagnosis of lack of environmental support to effect change in eating patterns evolved. The new plan will attempt to change the environment so that Mr. Smith can effect new dietary behaviors. The process demonstrates another analysis and a reorganization of assessment factors based on new data, leading to new nursing diagnoses to be tested. In this way more precise diagnoses are found that offer the client improved care and assistance.

CLIENT SITUATION: Mrs. Black

Mrs. Black is a 75 year old woman with the medical diagnosis of hypertension. She views health as the absence of disease and the need to take no medication. Two of her values are good health and the desire to maintain her medical regimen without fluctuations. In giving her history, she reports no headaches, dizziness, increase in dyspnea, orthopnea, paroxysmal nocturnal dyspnea, or pedal edema. She claims to be adhering to a low-salt diet. During the physical examination she was found to have a B.P. of 160/105, an H.R. of 88 and regular, with no murmurs, no JVD in an upright position, clear lungs, and no pedal edema. She does have an atrial gallop. She is obese: weight, 130 pounds; height $4'8''$. When speaking of discontinuing her medication she states, "I didn't take the extra methyldopa because it makes me so sleepy and I read about all those side effects. You know I don't like to take pills." At this time her body becomes tense, her eyes dart, and she speaks in staccato, terse statements. She fidgets in her chair. She reports eating sweets but not using any salt in cooking or at the table. Laboratory results revealed a normal SMA 12; serum sodium, 128 mEq/L; potassium, 3.5 mEq/L; chlorides, 102 mEq/L; and bicarbonate, 26 mEq/L.

---------------------------- NURSING DIAGNOSIS ----------------------------

Non-compliance secondary to fear of drugs (side effects), manifested by not taking her antihypertensive drugs.

Plan

For this nursing diagnosis, the plan is to promote compliance by providing an atmosphere that allows open discussion in regard to the taking of her antihypertensive medication.

Intervention

Nursing Interventions	*Outcome Criteria*
1. Focus on the clarification of feelings.	1. Client will discuss feelings and sources of feelings regarding her medications at first visit.

2. Discuss with client Becker's Health Belief Model, which states that the more a person sees himself as being vulnerable and health care treatment as being efficacious, the more compliant he will be. He then becomes ready to undertake compliant behavior.

2. Client will discuss motivation factors, susceptibility factors, vulnerability factors, extent of interferences with social roles, presence of symptoms, safety factors, efficacious factors, structural factors, attitudes, and enabling factors during the next three visits.

3. Have another health care professional validate need for and low risk of client's medication.

3. Client will listen to and ask questions of this other professional.

Evaluation

Evaluation demonstrated that Mrs. Black's compliance with drug therapy was not achieved by the interventions. She was slow to discuss feelings regarding her antihypertensive medication and had difficulty being specific about the source of these feelings. After discussion of factors from the Health Belief Model, Mrs. Black talked more about her feelings. She did not believe herself ill; she thought that the side effects of her medication and the change in her schedule were too costly and that the benefits did not compensate for these things.

Plan

For this same nursing diagnosis of non-compliance, the second plan is to offer alternate ways to decrease blood pressure.

Intervention

Nursing Interventions

1. Describe and practice relaxation technique.

2. Discuss 1000 calorie diet.

Outcome Criteria

1. Client will demonstrate the technique at every visit. Blood pressure will be less than 165/96 in one month.

2. Client will keep diet diary, and it will be discussed to determine its compliance with a 1000 calorie diet. Weight will be down one pound at the next visit.

3. Tell client to increase salt intake by using salt in cooking (because of slight decrease in serum sodium). Discuss relationship of high intake of sodium to hypertension and signs of fluid retention.

3. Client will verbalize relationship, list assessment factors for fluid retention, and maintain B.P. of less than 165/96.

4. Reorganize medication schedule to better accommodate client's schedule.

4. Client will discuss the improvement next visit. Blood pressure will be less than 165/96 in one month.

Evaluation

Evaluation demonstrated that the client did not lose weight, kept no diet diary, had no decrease in blood pressure, and did not practice the relaxation technique. She ran out of her medication once. She was able to verbally explain the diet, the relaxation method, and the need for medicine.

The interventions were not successful in this case. It was evident that Mrs. Black was not ready to comply with health suggestions. The second plan will be of no use until she views herself as "sick," sees benefit in taking medication, and sees the benefits of care as outweighing the costs of following the health suggestions.

The nursing diagnosis again provides for accountability. The interventions were unsuccessful because of an inaccurate nursing diagnosis based on incomplete assessment. New data need to be gathered to consider more complete nursing diagnoses for this hypertensive patient. Non-compliance is too broad. For more exact interventions, new diagnoses, *failure to see benefit of health care* and *failure to see self as sick* are to be explored. The plan is to clarify values and explore her feelings regarding the illness of hypertension and the benefits of medication. The outcome criterion will be that the client verbalizes her feelings until she sees the incongruities between her action and her needs. This plan will be instituted at the next visit.

CLIENT SITUATION: Ms. Sanchez

Ms. Sanchez, a 25 year old Puerto Rican woman, lives in a lower socioeconomic area of a large city. She is a single parent of four children ranging from two to twelve years of age. She is pursuing a college education as well as attempting to provide a supportive atmosphere for her children. She has a strained relationship with her boyfriend. She does not interact in a positive way with her mother, and she allows her mother to physically and verbally abuse her. Her medical diagnoses are hypertension and chest pain of unknown origin. Ms. Sanchez's concept of health is "being happy" and having "something good she knows is out there." Some of her values are that families are important, her children are important, and she is important.

The client expresses frustration with her children, with her living arrangements, and with her boyfriend. She wonders when she is going to "get a break for herself." She states that she wants to be a good mother, but she tires easily. She describes her chest pain as being left-sided, stabbing in nature, of sudden onset, and lasting 1/2 to 1 hour. It is relieved by 2 hours of rest. She is unaware of any precipitating or accompanying factors. She takes hydrochlorothiazide for her hypertension. She denies dyspnea on exertion, orthopnea, or paroxysmal nocturnal dyspnea.

During physical examination, the nurse sees a harried woman with two small children running around her. B.P. is 130/96; H.R. 78 and regular without murmurs or gallops; lungs are clear; no pedal edema; no JVD in an upright position. Client points with one finger to an area of chest pain at the nipple line of the left chest. Moderate exercise does not elicit any chest pain, disruption in rhythm, or abnormal changes in B.P.

Laboratory data show normal electrocardiogram, SMA 12, electrolytes, and chest x-ray.

The assessment suggested two nursing diagnoses:

1. Alteration in perceived locus of control secondary to feelings that she can't change her life and manifested by feelings of being manipulated, lack of self-confidence, and chest pain.

2. Strong drive toward self-actualization based on a verbalized strong self-concept and manifested by going to college and trying to offer her children a more supportive environment than she had.

NURSING DIAGNOSIS

Alteration in perceived locus of control secondary to feelings that she can't change her life and manifested by feelings of being manipulated, lack of self-confidence, and chest pain.

Plan

For the nursing diagnosis of alteration in perceived locus of control, the plan is to assist the client in clarifying and resolving conflicts, enhancing feelings of control and ability to cope, and lessening the need to use chest pain to cope.

Intervention

Nursing Interventions	Outcome Criteria
1. Use of nurse as a support, allowing patient to telephone nurse to discuss problems.	1. Client will telephone nurse at least once between visits to discuss problems and in 2 months all chest pain will subside.

2. Have client list priorities of problems.

2. Client will do so for second visit. She will discuss feelings about these problems at the next four visits and discuss ways to resolve them. Chest pain will also decline as conflicts resolve.

3. Discuss incongruities between client's verbal statements and behavior.

3. After 2 weeks client will begin to point out these incongruities between verbal statements and behavior.

4. Demonstrate step-wise problem solving techniques.

4. Client will begin using step-wise techniques at second visit.

5. Allow client to be angry and encourage her to handle her anger directly.

5. Client will start expressing anger at appropriate person after the second visit.

6. Support the client in making her own decisions.

6. Client will discuss problems and decisions with nurse.

Evaluation

Evaluation demonstrated that, at the end of two months, Ms. Sanchez was beginning to clarify and resolve conflicts. She could identify incongruities between her words and her behavior and was showing insights into who was deciding her behavior — herself or others. She was expressing anger more directly and making some decisions using a step-wise technique. She was having no chest pain. She decided to dissolve her relationship with her boyfriend and put firm limits on the relationship with her mother. She moved from her mother's residence. She described satisfactory relationships with all but one child, who was referred to a psychiatrist. The nurse continues to support the family while the child is in therapy.

NURSING DIAGNOSIS

Strong drive toward self-actualization based on a verbalized strong self-concept and manifested by going to college and trying to offer her children a more supportive environment than she had.

Plan

For this nursing diagnosis the plan is to support this drive and to foster her efforts to improve herself and her family.

Intervention

Nursing Interventions	*Outcome Criteria*
1. Refer to Family Services to request babysitting services.	1. Client will call Family Services by next visit.
2. Call churches to arrange for provision of food in emergencies.	2. Client will receive food in emergencies for herself and her children.
3. Refer to agency with free furniture and moving services.	3. Client will use these services if she needs them.
4. Provide recreational outlet.	4. Client will call the organization Parents without Partners.

Evaluation

Ms. Sanchez did obtain babysitting services, received extra food when necessary, and used the moving service. She verbalized an allowance of time for recreation. She did not choose to follow through with the club offered by the nurse practitioner. She continues at college, working with her children, and from time to time does part-time work.

CLIENT SITUATION: Mrs. Brown

Mrs. Brown, an obese 56 year old woman, arrived at the outpatient department with the medical diagnoses of angina, coronary atherosclerosis, and character disorder, which consists of life-long maladaptive patterns of behavior differing from neurotic or psychotic behavior. She values making her own decisions. Her friends are important to her because she is estranged from her family. She frequently is angry about the health care she receives from the doctors and the nurses.

She describes substernal chest pain, which occasionally radiates to the epigastric region and the left arm. At times it is relieved with rest or an antacid. It is sometimes aggravated by activity, certain foods, and emotional turmoil. She describes no pattern to the pain and a lack of understanding of how to relieve it. She smokes 1 to 2 packs of cigarettes per day, reports hypercholesterolemia, and does not exercise. She describes herself as friendly and outgoing most of the time but angry, depressed, lonely, and suicidal at other times. The medical doctor has prescribed nitroglycerin gr 1/150 for chest pain. Upon physical examination the nurse finds a woman, 5'3", weighing 160 pounds. B.P. is 136/80, H.R. 80 and regular with no murmurs or gallops, no JVD in an upright position, no pedal edema, and no organomegaly. Coarse rales (crackles) are found in the lungs; they change with coughing.

Serum cholesterol was found to be 350 mg per 100 ml. Coronary arteriography shows diffuse small vessel atherosclerosis that is inoperable. Stress test demonstrates depressed ST segment of 1 mm and heart rate of 130 causing chest pain.

The nursing diagnoses for Mrs. Brown were:

1. High risk for progressive coronary artery disease related to hypercholesterolemia, lack of exercise, psychological stress, smoking, and obesity, manifested by coronary atherosclerosis.

2. Knowledge deficit secondary to lack of health teaching, manifested by inability to distinguish cardiac chest pain from other types of chest pain.

3. Lack of preventive health action secondary to cost of compliance being higher than benefit acquired, manifested by anger at being told what to do and by non-compliance.

_____ NURSING DIAGNOSIS _____

High risk for progressive coronary artery disease related to hypercholesterolemia, lack of exercise, psychological stress, smoking, and obesity, manifested by coronary atherosclerosis.

Plan

For the nursing diagnosis of high risk for progressive coronary artery disease, the plan is to reduce the chance of coronary artery disease by decreasing cardiovascular risk-related factors.

Intervention

Nursing Interventions	Outcome Criteria
1. Promote weight loss and cholesterol reduction by:	1. Client will:
(a) clarifying feelings regarding diet.	(a) discuss feelings regarding diet the first two visits.
(b) securing two weeks of diet history.	(b) produce diet history the second and third visit.
(c) reorganizing eating habits using behavior modification.	(c) describe efforts to reorganize her eating behavior the third week.
(d) teaching diet low in cholesterol and low in calories.	(d) plan and use 1200 calorie low-cholesterol diet the fourth visit, and in one month client will start losing 1 to 2 pounds per week; cholesterol will decrease to 200 mg per 100 ml in two months.

(e) writing to welfare office to increase food stamp allotment to allow client to buy special foods.

(e) receive increased allotment from welfare office.

2. Encourage no smoking by supporting client in her efforts to reduce smoking gradually.

2. Client will have stopped smoking in four weeks.

3. Increase feelings of self-worth by:
   (a) exploring feelings of anger.

   (b) outlining her strengths and caring relationships.

   (c) giving her a prescription to say three times a day: "I'm a worthy person."

3. Client will:
   (a) describe feelings and sources of anger.

   (b) list her strengths and her caring relationships at the second visit.

   (c) report use of prescription at next visit and will describe two positive aspects about self in one month.

4. Outline walking programs by:
   (a) prescribing walking distances.

   (b) prescribing rate of increasing distances.

   (c) teaching pulse taking.

   (d) teaching signs and symptoms of complications.

4. Client will:
   (a) describe walking distance at every visit.

   (b) discuss distance increase at every visit.

   (c) demonstrate taking of own pulse at next visit.

   (d) discuss signs and symptoms at every visit.

Evaluation

On evaluation of Mrs. Brown's behavior, the nurse practitioner finds that the client is not losing weight, is not reducing her intake of cholesterol, is smoking, and is not exercising. She is voicing anger directly at the nurse, stating "... I don't need you to tell me what to do; I'll do it when I'm ready." She is making more positive statements about herself.

_____ NURSING DIAGNOSIS _____

Knowledge deficit secondary to lack of health teaching, manifested by inability to distinguish cardiac chest pain from other types of chest pain.

Plan

For the second nursing diagnosis the plan is to teach Mrs. Brown to distinguish between the many types of chest pain in order that she might act appropriately.

Intervention

Nursing Interventions	Outcome Criteria
1. Outline signs and symptoms of different types of chest pain such as that from ulcer, angina, hiatal hernia, lung disease.	1. Client will verbalize signs and symptoms of differing types of chest pain at every visit for three visits.
2. Describe use, action, and side effects of nitroglycerin; use of antacids; and position for client with hiatal hernia.	2. Client will use drugs and body positions correctly and report appropriate other symptoms to the nurse. Client will use emergency room for emergencies only.

Evaluation

Evaluation showed that Mrs. Brown takes nitroglycerin and antacids appropriately, reports important symptoms to practitioner, and has not used the emergency room indiscriminately.

In reviewing the appropriateness of the first nursing diagnosis, high risk for cardiovascular disease, the interventions were not successful. By reviewing the evaluation, the nurse feels the diagnosis is correct, but it needs to be paralleled by an additional nursing diagnosis:

_____ **NURSING DIAGNOSIS** _____

Lack of preventive health action secondary to cost of compliance being higher than benefit acquired, manifested by anger at being told what to do and by non-compliance.

Plan

Using the new diagnosis, the plan of action is to clarify the meaning of these life style changes to the client.

Intervention

Nursing Intervention	Outcome Criteria
1. Nurse will listen carefully and will encourage verbalization of feelings, particularly regarding changing of life style.	1. Client will clarify the meaning of her cardiovascular risk factors, will see incongruity between maintaining risk factors and attaining health, and will decide to change.

The making of the high risk diagnosis was difficult. Should each positive risk factor be a nursing diagnosis? A single positive factor carries less risk for a myocardial infarction. The danger results from the interaction of several risk factors. Therefore, the nursing diagnosis should reflect this interaction and does so by listing the positive factors under one diagnostic title.

CLIENT SITUATION: Mr. Green

Mr. Green is a 58 year old patient with medical diagnoses of chronic obstructive pulmonary disease, angina, peripheral vascular disease, and a history of diabetes mellitus. As a result of the diabetes, he has very poor vision. His concept of being healthy is to be physically active, for example, he likes to dance and to walk. His values are conservative. He believes that men are stoic, valiant, honest, strong, and protective of women. As a result of these views, he had some difficulty accepting the nurse as a practitioner at the beginning of the relationship. He was uncomfortable when the nurse was performing parts of the physical examination and discussing certain subjects. However, as the trust level of the nurse-client relationship increased, he became more at ease.

At present, he reports an infrequent cough with a small amount of white sputum production in the early morning. There has been no change in color of the sputum. His chest pain has not changed since his last visit. He describes an intense pain in the calves of his legs after walking two blocks on level ground. This is relieved with rest. He verbalizes anger and discouragement at not being able to control this pain. He is distressed at not "being what he used to be." For example, he states he can no longer dance, work, or even walk as far as he did in the past. Mr. Green smokes ten cigarettes per day.

On physical examination, the pulses in his extremities are weak. The lower extremities blanch upon elevation and remain so for 25 seconds after being lowered to the dependent position. Then they become very red. Toes have no hair; toenails are thick. Legs are very cool to the touch. No ulcers are present. Mr. Green demonstrates 20/200 vision using the Snellen chart. Mr. Green's facial expression is sad. His statements are those of resignation to his state of health. He has recently lost his pet, which he highly prized.

Laboratory data include normal fasting blood sugar and a high normal cholesterol level. Angiograms of the lower extremities show diffuse arteriosclerosis throughout all the small vessels, thereby negating the possibility of surgical bypass repair.

Three nursing diagnoses are suggested by the assessment data:

1. Hypoxia secondary to atherosclerosis, manifested by intermittent claudication.

2. Grief secondary to forced change in life style caused by chronic peripheral vascular disease and manifested by anger and discouragement.

3. Compliance secondary to trusting nurse-client relationship and his need to do "the right thing," manifested by his rigid adherence to a regimen.

_____ NURSING DIAGNOSIS _____

Hypoxia secondary to atherosclerosis, manifested by intermittent claudication.

Plan

For the nursing diagnosis of hypoxia, the plan is to maintain oxygenation of the extremities by decreasing the work demand of the extremities or increasing collateral circulation.

Intervention

Nursing Interventions	*Outcome Criteria*
1. Encourage his walking program to increase collateral circulation.	1. Client will maintain walking distance of at least six blocks every day, walking till pain occurs, then resting, then resuming walk.
2. Demonstrate leg exercises to increase collateral circulation.	2. Client will return demonstration at next office visit.
3. Outline methods of foot care and care of abrasions.	3. Client will return demonstration at next office visit. Feet will be dry, clean, and without abrasions; he will be wearing white socks and have his nails trimmed.
4. Smoking will be discouraged through discussions.	4. Client will smoke one less cigarette per day.
5. Dietary cholesterol intake will be reduced.	5. Client will report, through a diet history, eating three eggs a week, beef three times a week, use of margarine, and no use of butter. Serum cholesterol will remain normal.

Evaluation

Evaluation shows that Mr. Green has maintained his walking program and has at times exceeded the prescribed distances. He can return the leg exercise demonstration but admits doing the exercises irregularly at home. His diet history shows the recommended intake of fat but too many eggs. He has not decreased the number of cigarettes smoked. His serum cholesterol remains at a high normal level.

_____ **NURSING DIAGNOSIS** _____

Grief secondary to forced change in life style caused by chronic peripheral vascular disease and manifested by anger and discouragement.

Plan

In regard to the nursing diagnosis of grief, the plan is to assist the client with the grieving process and help him to find an alternative satisfying life style.

Intervention

Nursing Interventions	*Outcome Criteria*
1. Encourage verbalization of discouragement and frustration.	1. Client will discuss feelings regarding pain and immobility at every visit for six months.
2. Refer to Association for the Blind.	2. Client will have called the Association by the next visit.
3. Replace pet to give client something with which to exchange affection.	3. Client will have a new pet in three weeks.
4. Teach relaxation technique to decrease tension caused by loss of pet and to decrease pain.	4. Client will return demonstration next visit and describe decrease in pain.

Evaluation

Evaluation showed that Mr. Green was not able to perform the relaxation technique because of being "too nervous." He did verbalize frustrations. He does have a new pet, and he does communicate regularly with the Association for the Blind. Incorporating this evaluation into the ongoing nursing process, the nursing diagnosis remains the same, but the interventions will change. These interventions include (1) assisting Mr. Green with the technique every week until he can do it comfortably, and (2) supporting him with daily telephone calls until he can do it alone. An outcome criterion is that Mr. Green's nervous feelings will decrease.

_____**NURSING DIAGNOSIS** _____

Compliance secondary to trusting nurse-client relationship and his need to do "the right thing," manifested by his rigid adherence to a regimen.

Plan

In regard to the nursing diagnosis of compliance, the plan is for the nurse to be consistent in care in order to promote trust and compliance.

Intervention

Nursing Intervention	*Outcome Criteria*
1. Return all telephone calls; answer questions honestly; focus discussions on feelings every visit.	1. Client will continue to comply with medication and treatment regimens even as they change.

Evaluation

Mr. Green complied with most regimens, although there have been many changes caused by unsuccessful treatments.

SUMMARY

This chapter presented a variety of clients within an ambulatory care setting who received their primary health care from a nurse practitioner. The five-step nursing process model, with emphasis on nursing diagnosis, was utilized to illustrate the health care received by each client and the usefulness of the diagnosis to the practitioner. In addition, the chapter briefly addressed the role of a nurse practitioner in an ambulatory care setting.

References:

Becker, M., and Maiman, L.: Sociobehavioral determinants of compliance with health and medical care recommendations. *Medical Care*, *13*:10, 1975.

Berg, A.: Prevention in perspective. J. Family Practice, *9*:37, 1979.

Dunn, H.: High level wellness for man and society. *American Journal of Public Health*, *49*:786, 1959.

Robischon, P.: The public health nurse and chronic illness. *Nursing Clinics of North America*, *1*:433, 1966.

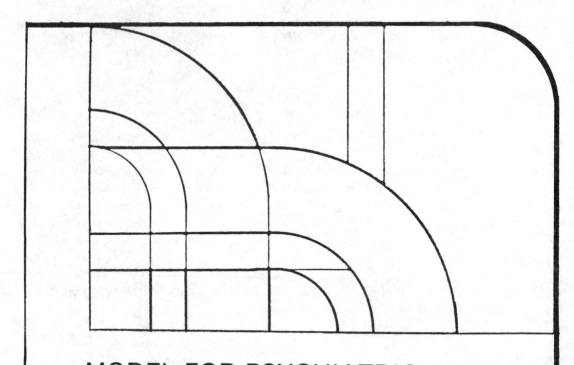

10 MODEL FOR PSYCHIATRIC AND MENTAL HEALTH NURSING: NEGATIVE SELF-CONCEPT

Ruth Beckmann Murray, R.N., M.S.N.

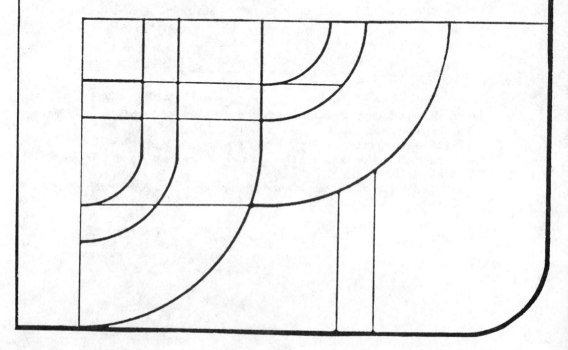

The nursing diagnosis, *negative self-concept*, is pertinent to many persons that the nurse cares for, since the person who is having difficulty adapting to stressors or crisis feels disorganized, helpless, and worthless. Often each member of a family with whom the nurse is working may have a negative self-concept, a feeling of "I'm not O.K."

This chapter will focus on the primary nursing diagnosis of negative self-concept in order to provide an in-depth analysis of the nursing diagnosis as it applies to emotionally ill clients. Regardless of the medical diagnosis — schizophrenia, depression, paranoia, neurosis, or the observable behaviors — most people who are given a psychiatric diagnosis will express negative feelings about the self. Usually the negative self-image and feelings about self have been present since early childhood. This negative self-concept affects the individual's ability to interact with others and, therefore, the ability to adapt to the interpersonal environment. Thus, the basis for emotional illness is formed.

A positive self-concept is basic to psychological adaptation. Psychological adaptation refers to the person's ability to achieve psychological integration and harmonious interpersonal relationships with the result that the person either changes his behavior in response to stimuli or changes the physical or social environment in order to better meet his needs. Adapting to the environment consists primarily of mastering at least some aspects of it, which contributes to the person's sense of self-worth and autonomy. If mastery cannot be accomplished, the adaptive person learns to accept difficulties and adjust as well as possible. The person has to come to terms with the environment because it affords the means by which basic needs can be met, but it also contains obstructions in the form of threats and pressures that interfere with meeting needs, create conflicting value systems, or hinder self-actualization.

Psychological stressors exist either in the real world or in the person's perception of a situation, and may come from either the external or internal environment. The person's individual perception of the event influences his reaction, which accounts for the variety of responses among people to a situation that objectively appears to be the same for all. Sometimes environmental stress is so great that the person's self-concept is threatened, and behavior becomes ineffective — frozen by anxiety. At other times the person's adaptation may be hampered because the environment lacks goods, services, and conditions that are necessary for adaptation and self-actualization (Studer, 1970). If the discrepancy between the person's goals and needs and environmental reality is too great, maladaption or dysfunction results; the person either becomes ill or tries to meet needs on a lower level of existence (Hall and Lindzey, 1970.)

Self-concept is the psychic representation or identity possessed by an individual, the central core of "I" around which all perceptions and experiences are organized. Self-concept is a dynamic combination of old and new experiences and includes the present feelings about self, physically, emotionally, and socially; expectations about the self; and perceptions of other's reactions to the self. The self-concept gives a sense of continuity and consistency to the person; it has a high degree of stability and represents

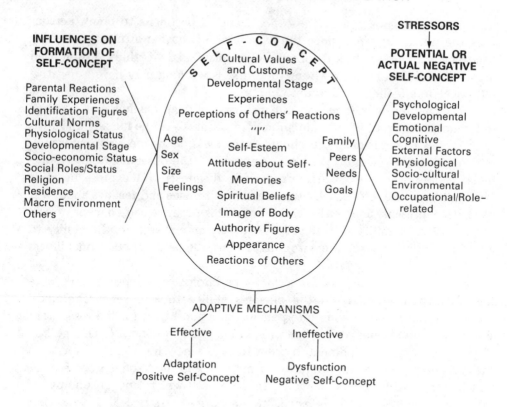

the person's fundamental frame of reference toward the self, either positive or negative. Self-concept is expressed through actions, words, intellect, attitudes, goals, and values (Coopersmith, 1967; Jacobsen, 1964; Roberts, 1978).

A major component of the self-concept is self-esteem. *Self-esteem is the evaluation that the person customarily maintains of himself and conveys to others by verbal reports or overt behavioral expressions.* This judgmental feeling about self includes a sense of approval or disapproval and indicates the extent to which the person believes himself capable, significant, successful, and worthy (Coopersmith, 1967). Self-esteem refers to the affirmation or acceptance of self because of basic worth, in spite of weakness or deficiency. The person who values self and feels valued by others usually has a positive self-concept; the person who feels worthless, does not feel respect from others, and does not respect himself usually has a negative self-concept.

Each person has numerous perceptions of self, based on sex, age, family role, occupational role, and use of leisure activity. Normally, these various facets or perceptions of the self, the various "masks" the person may wear when in different situations, are not too diverse or different from one another. A consistency remains even though the person feels differently about the self from time to time or is perceived in different ways by others. The psychiatric patient often has difficulty uniting the various facets of self into one image; he may not perceive the self with clarity, nor feel a sense of continuity, consistency, or stability.

Many factors influence the person's self-concept,* including:

1. Parental and others' reactions to the child's body and behavior from the time of birth and the reactions of others toward the person throughout life.

2. Norms of the culture or ethnic group, socio-economic background, and religion.

3. Family norms, values and relationships, family size, and birth order.

4. The person's interpretation of others' reactions to him.

5. Family attempts at class mobility and history of family geographic residence.

6. Anatomic appearance and physiological function of the body, including sex and age and kinesthetic and other sensorimotor stimuli.

7. Developmental stage of the person, including physical, emotional, and social maturation.

8. Attitudes and emotions regarding the self and the body, including body parts considered strategically important in the character of the ethnic or racial group, for example, the German backbone, Jewish nose, or black skin of the Negro.

9. Internal drives, dependency needs, and ideals to which the person aspires.

10. Identification with others who are considered ideal; a little of each significant person is incorporated into self-concept.

11. Roles, occupation, and various activities in which the person is involved.

12. Unity of memory, on which continuity of self is based.

*Blaesing and Brockhaus, 1972; Carlson, 1970; Coopersmith, 1967; Dempsey, 1972; Fisher, 1964; Murray, 1972 a,b; Simmel, 1966; and Wylie, 1961.

CASE STUDY

"Either you change your behavior or I'll fire you."

With the principal's words ringing in her ears, Mrs. K. frantically drove to the mental health clinic she had recently read about in the newspaper.

Mrs. K. was 48 years old, 5'4" tall, weighed 148 pounds, and appeared neatly dressed and groomed. She was a school teacher, and the past few months had been very difficult at school. Life had not been pleasant with her husband, Jim, and daughter, Kathy, for several years.

Mrs. K. was born in Omaha, Nebraska, the ninth of eleven children. In describing herself, she said: "I'm a dumb Polack." She described her mother as a "typical Polish mother — hardworking, stern, demanding obedience from the children, a devout Catholic, and too tolerant of the husband's faults." The family was very poor; the alcoholic father worked infrequently and most of the earnings were spent on liquor. Handouts and the meager earnings of her mother and the older children barely sustained the family. She flushed, and her voice became strident and angry as she described her early home life: her memories of the taunts from school children about her father, the beatings her mother and the children received from him, his favoritism toward the son, and her disgust with her mother for "putting up" with her father. She blamed the Catholic Church for allowing such a marriage to continue.

She remembered only a few pleasurable times during the elementary and high school years; the painful feelings of being an outcast and no good were recounted. She managed to receive above average grades in school in spite of her home conditions and general unhappiness.

After graduating from high school, she entered a religious order. The decision was not actually her own. Her mother had always wanted one of her daughters to be a nun. She assumed this role because none of the other six sisters had. Her family, except for one sister, supported her action, and one older married sister continued to send her essential supplies during her years in the convent.

Her 22 years as a nun were described angrily. She spoke of the constant stern and authoritarian attitudes of her supervisors, the harsh living environment, the general isolation from people, including the other nuns, the enforced humility, and the constant feelings of being no good and inferior. She was educated as an elementary teacher. She remembered disciplining the children harshly because her superiors told her to, but inside she felt such discipline was wrong. She remembered with affection and warmth only one rural parish to which she was sent. The two other nuns she had lived with were kind, the priest was amiable, she and the children were mutually fond of each other, and the parents were supportive. Apparently the mother superior felt she had been too friendly with everyone; she was moved after a year. Thereafter, she kept her emotional distance from everyone. She did the required work but little else.

For 22 years she endured what she described as loneliness, emptiness, reprimands, rigorous daily patterns of living, the inner anger and rebellion, and the constant sense of inferiority. Perhaps the social changes of the 1960's and early 1970's stimulated her decision; she left the order rather abruptly.

At the age of forty, with minimal social skills and no material goods, Mrs. K. re-entered the world. Her mother and siblings, except one, refused to talk to her; they felt disgraced. Only one sister, who was two years younger and had opposed her entry to the order, supported her decision and gave her some money and necessary supplies. Mrs. K. had maintained contact with two women who had left her order two years earlier. One lived in St. Louis, which influenced Mrs. K.'s decision to move there. This woman helped her buy clothes and introduced her to a hairdresser who not only fixed her hair but also extended friendship, helpful hints, and assistance with routine everyday problems.

The next two years were described as the happiest years of her life. She successfully taught fifth grade in a surburban school district, completed some courses toward her master's degree, joined a Catholic parish, and participated in the social activities of the church. She had fun at the dances for the single young adults in the church. One gentleman, a kind, quiet bachelor, was especially attentive. After a short courtship, he proposed marriage. She accepted, and in late August she became a bride.

In September, she continued teaching, and during the first month, her husband, ten years her senior, suffered a myocardial infarction. The physician declared him recovered and ready to return to work two months later. Mr. K. felt he could never work again; work might kill him. Thus, he applied for a pension from his place of employment but was unsuccessful in obtaining payment.

About this time Mrs. K. learned that she was pregnant. She stopped teaching at five-months gestation, as required by the district. Mr. K. was excited about having a child; Mrs. K. felt cheated, resentful, and angry. She felt she would now have two babies to care for — the child and Mr. K. He was demanding rather than attentive during the pregnancy.

When the daughter, Kathy, was born in May, Mrs. K. had no help. She felt inadequate as a mother and distant from the baby. Her husband, in spite of being home continually, did little to help. She did receive lots of advice from his family — his mother, two sisters, and a brother — who lived three blocks away. Somehow Mrs. K. got through the summer and the initial responsibility of child care. She realized at that time that she had never loved her husband; long ago the initial flattery of being chosen by another had worn off. Her inner anger formed a barrier between them. She was increasingly distant in her relationship to her husband and sexual relations occurred infrequently and only at his demand.

In September she returned to teaching, leaving the baby with her husband and in-laws. Mrs. K. was an effective teacher; her evaluations were excellent. She liked the principal, the other teachers, and the children. For the first time in her life she began to have some good feelings about herself — as a teacher. However, she continued to perceive herself as a bad person and mother.

After four years of teaching in one school, the district began to change in population distribution. She was placed in another school just three months prior to admission to the clinic. Events had gone from bad to worse: The fifth graders were inattentive and rowdy; the teachers seemed distant, not only from her but from each other; and the principal symbolized much of her earlier, but never forgotten, life. He flaunted authority, was threatening to the teachers, and was a harsh disciplinarian of the children. Since he was also a Free-Will Baptist minister, he frequently lapsed into sermon-like monologues during faculty meetings. Mrs. K. had felt demeaned and inferior from the first time she met him, and his 6'2" height and gruff voice reinforced her feelings.

For the three months prior to coming to the clinic, Mrs. K.'s negative feelings had magnified. She could no longer ignore feelings of being a bad person, worthless, and inferior when the work experience was unhappy. Her problem was compounded by the lack of support systems. She said she seldom attended church, had few friends, and the rift between her and her husband and daughter had grown wider. She was the breadwinner. She made the family decisions and talked very little to her husband. She nurtured her daughter the best she could, but Kathy was becoming more difficult to manage. Mr. K. and Kathy (now 4½ years old) spent a portion of most evenings and weekends with his family. Kathy usually got her way, in spite of Mrs. K.'s attempts to discipline her; she was learning how to manipulate all the family members as she gained independence and social skills. In fact, the situation at home and work had become so tense that recently Mrs. K. had thought of quitting her job and divorcing her husband, but she was ambivalent about what to do with Kathy. She had thought of suicide as a logical way to end everything.

Mrs. K. was unable to describe any specific suicide plans when asked. She replied, "I'm too stupid and inferior to even be successful at that, and anyway, I don't have enough courage."

Assessment

There was no pertinent past medical history; the client was referred for a complete physical examination to her own physician early in the counseling session. Mrs. K. reported that the physician found her overweight, but he had mentioned nothing else. Assessment of the adaptive status during initial sessions revealed the following information pertinent to the nursing diagnosis.

Psychological Adaptation: Emotional Status

1. Anxiety level moderate as indicated by:
    a. Rigid posture.
    b. Wringing hands and crying intermittently during sessions for the first month.
    c. Rapid, urgent speech; angry voice tone intermittently when describing past events that were emotion-filled; and crisp enunciation of words.
2. Mood mildly depressed for first three sessions.
3. Suicidal ideas stated at the first interview; thereafter, she insisted she was not contemplating suicide.
4. Ego functions intact:
    a. Oriented to time, person, and place.
    b. Reality contact maintained.
    c. Memory intact and extensive for recent and remote events.
    d. Sensory-perceptual functions unimpaired.
    e. Defense mechanisms primarily included
        (1) Rationalization for own behavior.
        (2) Projection of own inadequacy feelings onto husband.
        (3) Compensation: sarcastic remarks to other teachers and former nuns in an effort to overcome inferiority feelings.
        (4) Undoing: lack of home management skills were offset by meticulous housecleaning on Saturdays.

Plan of Care

The planning step of the nursing process involved formulating long- and short-term goals. Long-term goals and outcome criteria for determining their achievement are presented in Table 10–1. Short-term goals that contributed to achievement of the long-term goals and the desired result of therapy, a positive self-concept, are shown in Table 10–2.

Table 10–1 Long-Term Goals and Outcome Criteria

Long-Term Goals	Outcome Criteria
1. Develop more positive feelings about self and an identity and self-image of a self-actualizing, adaptive person.	a. Consistent realistic statements that describe self with positive adjectives. b. Demonstrated ability to change behavior in a positive or effective direction during stressful situations. c. Realistic positive statements about significant others. d. Initiation of at least one new activity that will be creative or challenging.
2. Establish happy and adaptive relationships with significant persons: family, friends, and work colleagues.	a. Consistent statements that are positive toward significant others. b. Daily harmonious conversation with husband and daughter, according to self-reports. c. Regular friendly conversations with work colleagues, according to self-reports. d. Weekly contact (direct or telephone) with at least 2 friends, according to self-reports. e. Consistent ability to speak with authority figures without feelings of intimidation or anger. f. Demonstrated ability to change own behavior in situations and to establish an environment that encourages others to change their behavior toward her.

Table 10–2 Short-Term Goals and Outcome Criteria

Short-Term Goals	Outcome Criteria
1. Express feelings of self-respect and self-acceptance.	1. State that decision to seek help was a sound one.
2. Verbalize anger.	2. Repeated statements of feeling less anger. Signs and symptoms of depression gradually reduced. State positive feelings about self. Behavior toward others increasingly adaptive.
3. Respond to rapport conveyed by nurse therapist.	3. Establish a nurse-client relationship.
4. Demonstrate increased sense of self-esteem. Feelings of inferiority reduced.	4. Try new behavior in interaction with others, becoming more adaptive.
5. Maintain a therapeutic relationship.	5. Statements indicate feeling accepted, in control of self, and trusting self and others. Make decisions. Respond more positively to others. Demonstrate new coping skills.
6. Improve interpersonal and social skills with family, work colleagues, and friends.	6. Be courteous to and talk and work with others in a positive, effective way. Report that others respond with positive feelings and maintain contact with her. Consistent adaptive behavior and statements reflecting strengthened sense of identity, trust, self-worth, and positive self-perceptions.
7. Clarify distorted perceptions of the principal, school children, her family, and others.	7. Clarified perceptions through talking and validating with an objective person. Deliberately choose adaptive behavioral strategies rather than reacting impulsively or habitually. Job performance and family relations improve.
8. Verbalize at least one positive, realistic statement at each therapy session.	8. Manifest positive self-concept. Report positive feedback from others. Engage in activities that are rewarding. Talk about accomplishments, feelings of achievement, independence, and self-confidence.
9. Terminate relationship. Demonstrate positive self-concept and maintain behavioral and attitudinal changes when three consecutive therapy sessions are scheduled at monthly intervals.	9. Talk about and work through feelings related to separation from a significant person. State feelings of independence and self-confidence about coping with future stresses. Review emotional, cognitive, and spiritual development. Demonstrate adaptive behaviors.

Short-Term Goals and Rationale

Short-term goals changed periodically throughout therapy, depending upon Mrs. K.'s behavior and verbal and non-verbal communication during the interview sessions. Table 10–2 shows the primary short-term goals and their outcome criteria. Although the goals are listed separately, often during intervention several of them would be utilized simultaneously. Table 10–2 also shows the progression of short-term goals from initiation to termination of professional help.

Intervention

The nurse who cares for people with psychological alterations of adaptation functions in a variety of nursing roles and may be responsible for physical care, technical procedures, a therapeutic milieu, health promotion measures, health teaching, and referral, in addition to counseling. One of the primary responsibilities of the nurse working with clients who suffer psychological alterations of adaptation is to establish and maintain a helping relationship through the use of effective communication and counseling skills, through insights about the developing person, and through a caring, empathic attitude and approach.

The helping relationship and measures used to facilitate a nurse-client relationship are the nursing intervention discussed in this chapter, since this is the primary intervention used with Mrs. K. in the clinic setting. Throughout the discussion, the term *nurse-therapist* is used interchangeably with *therapist*.

Establishment Phase

This phase of the relationship begins when the client seeks assistance or is brought for care. One of the responsibilities of the nurse is to carry out essential physical care measures for the client. However, to establish a relationship, the nurse must introduce herself, explain the nurse-therapist's role, and learn, through assessment, who the client is and what his expectations, health needs, and goals are. The client's role in the health care agency is reviewed. Together the nurse-therapist and client formulate a tentative care plan, and the therapist explains how the client and therapist will work together through a relationship (Peplau, 1952; Orlando, 1961; and Hofling, Leininger, and Bregg, 1967).

While the nurse is initially assessing the client, the client is also observing the nurse and may test the nurse with questions to determine if the nurse is trustworthy and interested in the client. During this phase, the client depends on the nurse. As the client feels more secure, he will disclose more of himself so that additional assessment data is gathered at each session during the establishment phase. During this assessment period, some intervention measures are also used (Peplau, 1952).

The first step in establishing a helping relationship with Mrs. K. was to establish *rapport, that is, creating a sense of harmony* through a warm friendly manner, appropriate smile, and eye contact. The following interventions are involved in establishing rapport:

1. Relate to the other as an equal to eliminate social barriers, convey acceptance, and promote a sense of trust.

2. Find a common interest or experience for initiating conversation.

3. Establish a smooth, easy pattern of conversation.

4. Convey a keen, sympathetic interest in the other person, give full attention, listen carefully, and indicate that there is plenty of time.

5. Adopt another's terminology and conventions and meet him on his own ground to the extent possible (Argyle, 1967).

Trust is essential to any helping relationship. *Trust is the firm belief in the honesty, integrity, reliability, and justice of another person without fear of outcome.* Mrs. K.'s experiences with people had not always been based on trust. Thus, a trusting relationship depended upon the attitude, flexibility, consistency in response, maturity, and reliability of the nurse-therapist. Mrs. K. could not share important personal information if she could not rely on the therapist and feel sure that the therapist would react with the same behavioral characteristics each time. A sense of confidentiality was also maintained. A sense of mutual trust was established within a few sessions and was maintained throughout therapy. Mrs. K. was seeking help and was responsive to the caring manifested by the therapist (Rogers, 1951).

Because of Mrs. K.'s negative feelings toward self, unconditional positive regard and acceptance were conveyed by the therapist throughout therapy. *Unconditional positive regard is the demonstrated belief in the dignity, worth and importance of the person, regardless of his behavior.* The therapist demonstrates this attitude by reaching out, by learning about the uniqueness of the person, and by being willing to stimulate a more likable behavior in the person. *Acceptance means interest in and concern for another because he is a human being with dignity, and it includes avoiding moralistic judgment and expressions of shock or disapproval at the person's behavior or statements. It also includes conveying to another person that he is worth all of the attention, skill, energy, and understanding that he needs.* Acceptance does not mean that the therapist insists on changing the client's behavior, but rather that the therapist is willing to assist the client when he is ready to change (Rogers, 1951).

Unconditional positive regard and acceptance cannot be fully conveyed until the client's unique characteristics are better known by the therapist. However, the therapist who has a positive self-concept and self-acceptance has the emotional energy to convey positive feelings toward the client.

Empathy, feeling with the person, understanding her behavior, and being motivated to act on the client's behalf, is another essential characteristic for establishing a helping relationship (Rogers, 1951). Empathy enables the therapist to sense the client's private world and her feelings as if they belonged to the therapist, without losing the "as if" quality, so that the therapist's feelings do not get bound up in the interaction. Empathy is possible to the degree that the therapist can abstract from personal life experiences, by way of recall or generalization, common factors that are applicable to the client's problems. Statements that served as an emotional mirror or as a reflection of feeling told Mrs. K. that she was understood, and such statements encouraged her to delve deeper into her own memories and share more of her own feelings and experiences. As she gained courage to examine her feelings and experiences and their underlying origins and distortions, Mrs. K. gained new self-understanding. Gradually, she became free to change her behavior, that is, to try more adaptive behavior with other people.

During this phase, effective interviewing techniques were used to assist Mrs. K. in describing problems, needs, and expectations, and in actively participating in setting goals.

Identification Phase

This phase has been compared developmentally to the childhood phase. During the period of interaction, the client responds selectively to the person who seems to offer the needed assistance. The therapist is perceived by the client as accepting, congruent, trustworthy, and empathic and becomes the client's identification figure (Hofling, Leininger, and Bregg, 1967). This is the phase during which the therapist and client become better acquainted as they mutually explore the client's deeper feelings, needs, and goals. He trusts the therapist's decisions and actions, works closely with the therapist, follows suggestions, and often claims that the therapist "has all the answers." The therapist becomes an ego ideal for the client and must be able to tolerate the client's dependency (Hofling, Leininger, and Bregg, 1967).

Developmental progress results when the client is able to identify with some of the healthy characteristics of the therapist. As the sense of trust deepened, Mrs. K. began to show signs of the identification phase of the relationship. She listened closely to the therapist, repeated key interpretive statements, and tried to act between sessions on the suggestions given to her.

She became motivated to continue to talk, to learn about herself, to change her perspective of herself and others, and to change her behavior. She utilized the strengths conveyed to her non-verbally and verbally by the therapist. She remained very much a unique individual but she utilized the therapist as a role model.

The identification phase involves *transference, whereby the client unconsciously displaces onto or invests in the therapist the patterns of behavior and emotional reactions that originated with childhood, especially with parents* (MacKinnon and Michels, 1971). Mrs. K. had deep unresolved feelings about her past authority figures. She first saw the therapist as an authority figure. But the therapist did not respond like the authority figures in her past or like the present authority figure, the school principal. Therefore, Mrs. K. was able to talk through angry feelings about authority, try new behavior with the authority figure, and learn that not all authority figures act in the same preconceived way. She began to act more like an authority figure with Kathy, assuming a more active role as a parent by trying some of the ideas suggested by the therapist.

Working or Therapeutic Phase

Developmentally, this phase is similar to adolescence. During this phase the client becomes more independent and uses all of the services and resources offered by the therapist that meet his needs. The client becomes more assertive and self-reliant as he tries self-care measures, insists on doing things his own way, or tries more adaptive ways of behaving with others. The client's increased self-esteem and positive self-image are apparent as he talks, initiates action, and analyzes his behavior and its effects. During this phase the therapist facilitates behavioral change, helps the client work through problems at his own pace, offers support and hope, and promotes insight to the greatest degree possible. The additional learning that is acquired by the client promotes use of new coping skills and adaptation (Peplau, 1952; Orlando, 1961; and Hofling, Leininger, and Bregg, 1967).

Acceptance, positive and warm feelings, trustworthiness, and empathy were conveyed, and purposeful communication methods were continued with the client throughout this phase of the nurse-client relationship. The caring and sense of responsibility for Mrs. K. deepened as the therapist gained more knowledge about her as a unique person. Mrs. K. was hurting emotionally but was also trying to become developmentally more mature and adaptive.

Purposeful communication (Greenhill, 1956; Hays and Larson, 1963; and Peplau, 1952 and 1964) involved careful listening to Mrs. K.'s total message rather than selective listening to the parts that were obvious, that met the therapist's preconceived ideas, or that were enjoyable or easy. The diagnosis of depression with suicidal ideas would have been too confining to structure the therapy sessions and relationship. Rather than putting a diagnostic label on Mrs. K., the therapist tried to look at Mrs. K. and her world from Mrs. K.'s perspective. Careful listening to the history she recounted helped the therapist to feel with Mrs. K. her very low self-regard and her sense of inferiority and lack of worth that structured how she responded to others and influenced others' responses to her.

Effective interviewing techniques were used during the entire intervention step of the nursing process. Open-ended, indirect questions encouraged Mrs. K. to talk about the feelings and ideas that were important to her at that particular session. Related questions were asked not only to gain additional understanding on the therapist's part but also to help Mrs. K. put her life history into a logical sequence, to clarify her feelings, and to gain a new perspective on her own or another's behavior. The therapist stated the feelings that were implied by Mrs. K.'s non-verbal behavior in order to encourage her to describe feelings and to accept them as a valid part of herself. Reflecting or restating helped Mrs. K. analyze in greater depth her motivations and the effects of her behavior.

Basic to the use of purposeful communication techniques was the therapist's ability to *make positive statements* to Mrs. K. about her appearance, motivation to change, attempts at more effective behavior on the job and in the home, and efforts at resuming friendships or in trying new activities. Continual positive reinforcement that was realistic was given even in the first session: Mrs. K. was told that her seeking of help was a sign of her ability to think things through logically and to act on her own behalf. Thereafter, the therapist always found at least one aspect of Mrs. K. and her behavior to comment on favorably. Mrs. K. at first verbally minimized these positive statements, but because positive feedback was *consistently* and *honestly* given, she gradually introjected these statements into her self-concept.

Promoting expression of angry feelings was an early goal and was begun at the second session through careful use of communication techniques. Anger had been repressed for most of her life; it took many sessions to work through her anger and be rid of past angers. The therapist at first had to tell Mrs. K. that she sensed Mrs. K. felt upset and very angry about all of the unhappy events in her life, present and past, and that it was all right to talk about these feelings. When Mrs. K. realized that the therapist would listen and accept her — anger and all — Mrs. K. talked without stopping for one-half hour. Words and feelings tumbled out together. For many sessions, whenever an emotionally loaded subject came up, the tirade of anger would come forth. Many of the negative feelings that Mrs. K. described were directed against herself, but she also spoke negatively of the other persons and events in her present and past life. She had suffered many deprivations and losses and needed to resolve her feelings.

The therapist listened, waited patiently for her to phrase her thoughts, validated that her feelings were normal, and did not take the anger personally. Issues or events behind the angry feelings were explored. The therapist remained calm and supportive and reinforced Mrs. K.'s ability to be honest about her feelings. Ways to more effectively express anger that she felt toward others were explored for many sessions. Mrs. K.'s ideas on how she felt she could overtly show her interest in others were explored. Suggestions were made by the therapist on ways to re-establish relations with family, work colleagues, and friends.

The principles of catharsis and reinforcement of appropriate behavior can work effectively over a period of time. The therapist reinforced Mrs. K.'s expression of feelings by continuing to invite her statements and to listen. As the anger lessened, the therapist explored ways in which she could better meet her needs. The therapist recognized verbally her attempts to change behavior and to look at self and others in a new way. Concern and assistance can motivate the client to try new behavior, and as Mrs. K. saw results and felt better about herself, she became motivated from within to continue more adaptive behavior.

Part of Mrs. K.'s sense of inferiority and anger was related to her strict super ego, her high ideals and aspirations, her strict standards for what she should be able to do, and her desire "to be perfect." She blamed herself for not living up to her standards and also blamed others for her lack of achievement. Again, the self-deprecation was listened to, and others were not defended as she made accusatory remarks. By helping her to develop a realistic time and sequential perspective of her major life events, Mrs. K. could gradually gain a sense of control over the happenings of her life. Cause and effect were related when appropriate. She sometimes repeated some of the same story in several sessions; this was accepted to allow for thorough catharsis and resolution of feelings. After one or two descriptions of an event, the feelings of loss, rejection, deprivation, and anger would be discharged and blame of others or self was no longer necessary. The therapist encouraged her self-understanding through clarification of the situation and feelings and explanation or interpretation of the dynamics involved. The therapist consistently reinforced the idea that Mrs. K's ability to explore painful situations and feelings was a sign of gaining control over her own behavior and a new sense of self or identity. Mrs. K. was maturing, and it was important to help Mrs. K. realize what she was accomplishing. The therapist also helped her gain a realistic picture of her strengths and limits; such statements and explanations had to be repeated many times in order to help Mrs. K. to adjust her standards and to internalize her strengths and accept them as part of herself. Recognition of her accomplishments and her many likable personality traits was repeated. Acceptance of Mrs. K's limits and failures by the therapist and validation that these were a part of being human helped Mrs. K. to accept her own limits.

Spiritual aspects must be considered in intervention. Because she felt alienated from her church and God, the therapist spoke of God's love and care for her. Mrs. K. was encouraged to talk to her friends who were formerly nuns about spiritual matters as a first step. Because she disliked the priest of her parish, she was encouraged to explore spiritual ideas and feelings with the therapist until she could contact another priest who had been helpful to her in the past. Both the therapist and the other spiritual leaders had to convey an agape love for Mrs. K. to help her feel like a unique person and a child of God who could be forgiven, who could forgive others, who was lovable, and who could extend love to others.

Although Mrs. K. was a low risk for suicide, the therapist used the *supportive, warm relationship as a deterrent to suicidal ideas.* By telling Mrs. K. that she was important to herself, her family, and her friends, by conveying acceptance of her as a unique person, and by exploring ways that Mrs. K.'s life situation could improve, the therapist helped Mrs. K. to believe that life held promise for her. As she began to feel better about herself, she wanted to live to raise Kathy. Then, gradually, she also wanted to live in order to restructure her relationship with her husband, her own family, her friends, and her work colleagues. Gradually, she even came to accept her in-laws, although she could not establish close ties with them.

Termination Phase

This phase of the nurse-client relationship is marked by the client becoming as fully adaptive and independent as possible. Previously unmet needs have been resolved or met, goals have been accomplished, and the client is ready to be discharged from the health care system. This phase is likened developmentally to adulthood. The main issue to be explored in this phase are the feelings related to loss and separation as the client is freeing himself from the therapist and is mobilizing strength and ability to stand alone. The therapist and client explore his illness and its meaning to him, his strengths and adaptive skills, his changed self-concept, and his ability to manage in the future. Discharge and teaching plans are reviewed and integrated into the client's life-style as appropriate. The therapist reaffirms that the relationship has been meaningful and can serve as a basis for future relationships (Peplau, 1952, Orlando, 1961; Hofling, Leininger and Bregg, 1967).

Preparation for termination must be planned by the therapist and must begin months ahead of discharge. Therapy sessions were initially scheduled weekly. When Mrs. K. was able to maintain realistic positive feelings and ideas about herself and initiate different kinds of behavior with the significant people in her environment between sessions, therapy was scheduled for alternate weeks, and then for once every three weeks. The last three sessions were scheduled at monthly intervals. As she maintained the ability to make insightful interpretations of some of her own behavior, to describe understanding of others' behavior, to utilize the interpretations made by the therapist, and to act on these interpretations, scheduling therapy less frequently was another way to convey that she was seen as an increasingly healthy, mature person, and was preparing for termination of the nurse-client relationship. Preparation for termination was made gradually so that loss of the relationship could be resolved. Feelings of separation, the meaning of the relationship to both Mrs. K. and the therapist, and how Mrs. K. would continue to manage were explored over several sessions. Mrs. K. had re-established and tightened relationships with her daughter, husband, friends, her sisters and their families, and even her mother, and these ties plus her improved working relationships meant that she had used the therapist's support and the helping relationship in an effective way. After eighteen months she had no further need for therapy.

In summary, the interventions carried out by the nurse-therapist in order to help Mrs. K. to accomplish her short- and long-term goals included:

1. Establishing rapport and trust.

2. Conveying acceptance and empathy.

3. Using therapeutic communication and effective interviewing techniques.

4. Encouraging ventilation of anger.

5. Using interventions to prevent suicide.

6. Giving positive reinforcement to her behavior frequently, as appropriate.

7. Establishing and maintaining a therapeutic nurse-client relationship.

8. Encouraging her interpretation of behavior and feelings.

9. Presenting courses of action and ideas on how to better cope with situations and how to change behavior to be more adaptive (job, husband, daughter, friends, housework, activity, hobbies, and so on).

10. Validating her appropriate interpretations, ideas, behavior, and choices of alternatives.

11. Summarizing her progress in behavior and her improving self-image when appropriate.

12. Encouraging mutual evaluation of progress.

13. Terminating the relationship.

Evaluation

In the nursing situation just described, the evaluation steps of the nursing process must include (1) determining whether outcome criteria were achieved by the client by the time of discharge and (2) determining the effectiveness of the therapist's approach with the client. While this step is discussed last, evaluation must follow intervention measures, or intervention to promote psychological adaptation is unlikely to be effective.

Research by Carl Rogers (1951) and others indicates that it is primarily the self-concept that changes during effective client-centered therapy. The person becomes less demanding of self and others, and overall behavior and achievement improves. The person appears better adjusted and describes a greater degree of inner content, self-understanding, self-acceptance, and self-value, and displays greater self-responsibility. The person after therapy expresses greater satisfaction with self and others and greater comfort in relationships with others. The person makes choices and establishes values differently, and meets frustration with less prolonged physiological tension and with more adaptive emotional and behavioral responses. He behaves in ways that are less defensive, less infantile, and more socialized and is more accepting of reality in self and in the social environment. The person becomes more adaptive and improves in problem-solving ability.

Mrs. K. demonstrated such behavioral changes during the course of therapy. She became more adaptive, and in turn, others changed toward her. This encouraged her to continue to work out her negative feelings, to develop new social skills, and to establish closer ties with others.

Short-term goals numbered 1, 2, and 3 in Table 10-2 were initial goals that were essential for goals numbered 4 and 5 to be met. Goal number 5, establishing a nurse-client relationship, was met after the third or fourth therapy session, since Mrs. K.'s interpersonal needs were strong, although her overt behavior created distance between her and others. The therapeutic relationship deepened over time, as would be expected. Goals numbered 1, 2, 4, 6, 7, and 8 guided intervention at every therapy session; these goals contributed to maintenance of a nurse-client relationship and Mrs. K.'s increasing adaptation.

During the Establishment Phase in intervention, Mrs. K. learned to trust the therapist, and as the relationship moved through the Identification and Working Phases, she learned to trust herself and then others. Her suicidal ideas were dropped after the initial sessions; her complaints and appearance of depression were diminished shortly thereafter. As the therapist became better acquainted with Mrs. K. and as the relationship moved into the

Identification and Working Phases, the therapist gave positive reinforcement to Mrs. K. whenever it was appropriate. Mrs. K. responded to the warmth, positive feelings, and acceptance that were conveyed non-verbally and verbally, but internalization of positive feelings into her self-concept and adaptive changes in personality took many sessions. Identification with the therapist gradually enabled Mrs. K. to act on the positive statements. As she changed her behavior in a positive direction, others around her noticed the change and responded accordingly. The process was slow; at times her behavior seemed to regress for a week or two. But over a period of time, the attempts at autonomy, self-control, and increased adaptability with others, even in the face of stress, elicited new responses from others, which reinforced flexibility and new responses in her. Simultaneously, but slowly, she changed her feelings about herself. Over a year elapsed before she really believed she was a good, competent person of worth and dignity, but each time she made an insightful statement about her own or other's behavior and each time she identified a positive characteristic or action within herself, she was one step closer to a positive self-concept.

During the Working Phase of the relationship, Mrs. K. was able to work through feelings of hate and anger directed toward past and present authority figures. Gradually, blaming also diminished; she learned how her angry feelings and behavior, however covert, alienated her from others and caused others to reject her. As she became more realistic in her perspectives about herself, what she was, and her strengths and limits, she became less demanding that others be perfect. Her statements about herself and her behavior conveyed that she saw herself as a worthwhile, competent, lovable person and that she felt love and concern for others. She initiated new hobbies for herself and activities with others.

When adaptive strategies were maintained, and the long-range goals were demonstrated, goal number 9, termination of the relationship, was accomplished in three sessions scheduled at monthly intervals. However, preparation for termination began earlier.

During the Termination Phase, Mrs. K. was accomplishing the developmental tasks of generativity relevant to a mature woman in mid-life (Erikson, 1964). The long-term goals had been reached, and the evaluative criteria were demonstrated by Mrs. K. She had developed more positive feelings about self and an identity and self-image of a self-actualizing, adaptive person. Happy and adaptive relationships with family, friends, and colleagues at work had been established.

Evaluation by the therapist of her approach to the client was ongoing. At the end of each session throughout therapy, the therapist reviewed her notes taken during the session to determine if effective communication methods had been used and if the main verbal and non-verbal messages had been responded to. Feelings conveyed by Mrs. K. were examined, and the therapist also examined her own feelings and responses to Mrs. K. and the session. Periodic meetings with a supervisor also helped the therapist to validate feelings and therapy approaches. Communication and relationship measures used during intervention were effective. The therapist's self-awareness served as a basis for promoting the client's self-awareness. Therapy with Mrs. K. had been a rewarding experience.

References:

Argyle M.: *The Psychology of Interpersonal Behavior*. Baltimore, Penguin Books, 1967.

Blaesing, S., and Brockhaus, J.: The development of body image in the child. *Nursing Clinics of North America, 7:* 597, 1972.

Carlson, C. (ed.): *Behavioral Concepts and Nursing Intervention*. Philadelphia, J.B. Lippincott Company, 1970.

Coopersmith, S.: *The Antecedents of Self-Esteem*. San Francisco, Freeman Publishing Company, 1967.

Dempsey, M.: The development of body image in the adolescent. *Nursing Clinics of North America, 7:*609, 1972.

Erikson, E.: *Childhood and Society*, 2nd ed. New York, W.W. Norton & Company, Inc., 1964.

Fisher, S.: Sex differences in body perception. *Psychological Monographs, 78:*1, 1964.

Greenhill, M.: Interviewing with a purpose. *American Journal of Nursing, 56:*1259, 1956.

Hall, C., and Lindzey, G.: *Theories of Personality*, 2nd ed. New York, John Wiley & Sons, Inc. 1970.

Hays, J., and Larson, K.: *Interacting with Patients*. New York, Macmillan Publishing Company, 1963.

Hofling, C., Leininger, M., and Bregg, E.: *Basic Psychiatric Concepts in Nursing*, 2nd ed. Philadelphia, J.B. Lippincott Company, 1967.

Jacobsen, E.: *The Self and the Object World*. New York, International Universities Press, Inc., 1964.

MacKinnon, R., and Michels, R.: *The Psychiatric Interview in Clinical Practice*. Philadelphia, W.B. Saunders Co., 1971.

Murray, R.: Body image development in adulthood. *Nursing Clinics of North America,* 7:617, 1972. (a)

Murray, R.: Symposium on the concept of body image — forward. *Nursing Clinics of North America,* 7:593, 1972. (b)

Orlando, I.: *The Dynamic Nurse-Patient Relationship*. New York, G.P. Putnam's Sons, 1961.

Peplau, H.: *Interpersonal Relations in Nursing*. New York, G.P. Putnam's Sons, 1952.

Peplau, H.: *Basic Principles of Patient Counseling*, 2nd ed. Philadelphia, Smith, Kline & French Laboratories, 1964.

Roberts, S.: *Behavioral Concepts and Nursing Throughout the Life Span*. Englewood Cliffs, N.J., Prentice-Hall, Inc., 1978.

Rogers, C.: *Client Centered Therapy*. Boston, Houghton, Mifflin Company, 1951.

Simmel, M.: Developmental aspects of the body scheme. *Child Development,* 37:83, 1966.

Studer, R.: The dynamics of behavior — contingent physical systems. *In* Preshansky, H., Setlson, W., and Riulin, L.: *Environmental Psychology: Man and his Physical Setting*. New York, Holt, Rinehart & Winston, Inc., 1970.

Wylie, R.C.: *The Self-Concept: A Critical Survey of Pertinent Research Literature*. Lincoln, University of Nebraska Press, 1961.

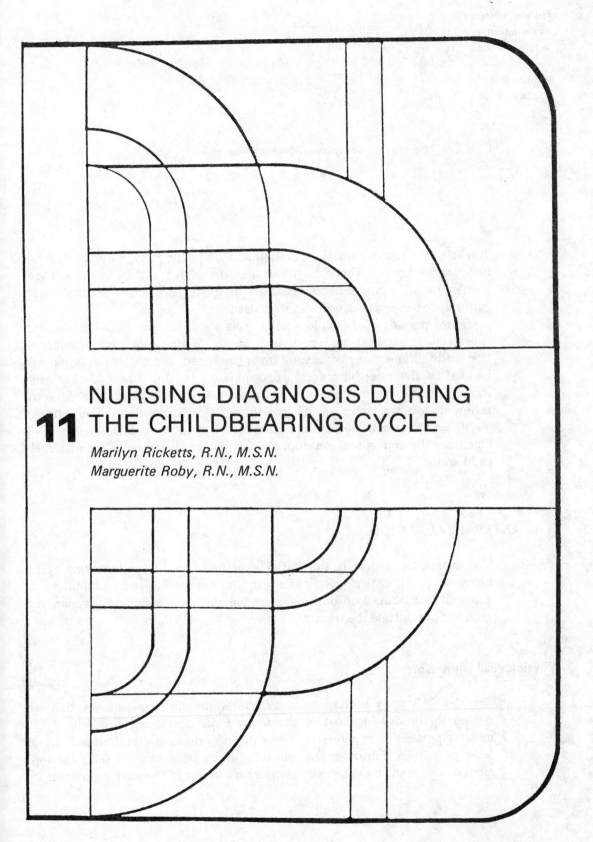

11 NURSING DIAGNOSIS DURING THE CHILDBEARING CYCLE

Marilyn Ricketts, R.N., M.S.N.
Marguerite Roby, R.N., M.S.N.

History, physical examination, and laboratory data focusing on mother-child health care needs	→	Extrapolation of significant data and use of pertinent knowledge	→	Nursing Diagnosis

Figure 11-1 Development of nursing diagnosis.

This chapter focuses on the development of nursing diagnoses during the childbearing cycle. These diagnoses are formulated within the theoretical framework of adaptation as reflected in its physiological, psychological, cultural, developmental, and social dimensions.

Three periods of the childbearing cycle are discussed in this chapter: the antepartal, intrapartal, and postpartal period. Within each period, information on the dimensions of adaptation is presented, and a client example will be used to illustrate the process of formulating nursing diagnoses. For each client, the nursing history, physical examination, and laboratory data are reviewed for the purpose of presenting significant data. The nursing diagnoses are formulated from aggregates of significant data. Figure 11-1 illustrates the conceptual development of nursing diagnosis in the maternal-child area.

THE ANTEPARTAL PERIOD

The antepartal period is the initial experience in the childbearing cycle; hence it is of critical importance to mother and fetus. Adaptation is demanded of both in an ongoing sequence of events designed to prepare the fetus for life outside the uterus.

Physiological Dimension

The mother's body undergoes many alterations during pregnancy that are related to the development of the fetus. Fetal development is one of the most important parameters to assess during pregnancy, and alterations in fetal growth are followed very carefully. Such assessment of fetal development can be made by externally measuring the size of the growing uterus.

Closely related to fetal growth is maternal nutrition. The mother provides nutrition for fetal development. It is important for the expectant mother to have an adequate protein intake along with iron and folic acid for the biosynthesis of red blood cells. In many instances, the diet of the mother can be directly correlated with fetal outcome. It is necessary, therefore, for the nurse to identify any alterations in nutrition (Higgins, 1972).

The nurse should be aware of optimal patterns of weight gain during pregnancy and of variations in weight gain. Weight changes should be plotted at each prenatal visit and the reason for the change investigated. In some cases it may be related to an inadequate diet. In other cases, it may be related to a disease process. For example, a symptom of pre-eclampsia is a rapid weight gain in the third trimester of pregnancy.

Maternal metabolism undergoes many complex biochemical alterations during pregnancy. Glucose consumption is altered by hormonal changes of pregnancy. The cells become more resistant to the effects of insulin, creating a relative glucose intolerance. For this reason it is important to check the urine for the presence of glucose throughout pregnancy.

Assessment of the fetal-placental unit is very important for identifying complications of pregnancy. In the first trimester of pregnancy, bleeding or abdominal cramping may be a sign of impending abortion. Bleeding during the third trimester of pregnancy may point to an alteration in the functioning of the placenta as in placenta previa and abruptio placentae. It is also very important to assess fetal heart tones at each prenatal visit. Alterations of the fetal heart rate outside the normal range of 120 to 160 may indicate fetal complications. If a baby is overdue past 40 weeks gestation, the assessment of the fetus assumes greater significance because the aging placenta becomes a less effective organ of perfusion for oxygen, nutrients, and removal of wastes. Alterations in fetal-placental functioning is only one of the areas from which nursing diagnoses may be developed during the antepartal period.

Some of the normal physiological alterations that occur during pregnancy create minor discomforts for the mother. Nausea and vomiting, two of the most common complaints during the first trimester of pregnancy, are probably associated with alterations in hormonal and gastrointestinal functions during the first trimester of pregnancy (Clausen and coworkers, 1976). Many pregnant women complain of backaches. These are associated with changes in body balance related to the increasing size and weight of the gravid uterus, which places a strain on the spinal column and the muscles supporting the torso. Many other minor discomforts of pregnancy are reported, and it is important that the pregnant woman understand the causes of these discomforts and the methods to relieve them.

Environmental factors are important to assess, since they may deleteriously affect the physiological adaptive ability of the fetus. Smoking during pregnancy may alter the birth weight of the fetus, resulting in a small-for-gestational-age fetus. If the mother consumes alcohol during the pregnancy, fetal alcohol syndrome may result. Environmental hazards may also yield nursing diagnoses during the antepartal period.

Psychological Dimension

Psychological adaptation is affected by the many changes that pregnancy causes. Alterations in body image occur during pregnancy because of rapid changes in the body (Iffrig, 1972; Fawcett, 1978). Some women react to the change in their body very favorably, while other women may be threatened by these changes. Body image is related to the individual's self-concept and her attitude toward her pregnancy. It is important to promote a positive sense of self in the pregnant woman (Rubin, 1970; McConnell and Daston, 1961). If the mother and father have a positive attitude toward the pregnancy and desire a child, it will be easier for them to resolve the crisis that pregnancy brings. Pregnancy causes a certain amount of disequilibrium as the family members utilize their resources to come to grips with their feelings about the pregnancy, future childbearing, and childrearing (Olds and coworkers, 1980).

Social Dimension

Pregnancy often creates a disruption in the mother's career. Many women who have enjoyed a career and who find the idea of giving it up very unsatisfactory may elect to continue their career. This often creates role overload for the new mother until she is able to adjust to the demands of her new baby and the demands of her career and home. For the mother who has elected to give up her career, she may have many feelings of loss until she becomes adjusted to her new lifestyle.

Cultural Dimension

Understanding the cultural components of a client's background helps the nurse to understand the behavior of her client, and to individualize her care. Culture affects a woman's attitude toward her pregnancy. It also influences the mother's behavior during labor and delivery, the amount of bedrest she takes after birth, the type of care she seeks, the care she gives her infant, and the method she will choose to feed her baby (Clark and Affonso, 1979; Anderson, 1974).

Developmental Dimension

Pregnancy itself is considered to be a developmental task, and the chief milestones are confirming the pregnancy, accepting the pregnancy, realizing the fetus is a separate individual, the birth of the baby, and the development of attachment to the baby (Caplan, 1970).

Duvall (1971) identifies the period of pregnancy and childbirth as a developmental stage in the expanding family that parallels the individual's development. It seems reasonable to assume that the more adjusted and psychosocially mature individual will be better prepared to cope with the crisis of pregnancy. If the individuals are prepared to give of their time and of themselves for the goal of childrearing, they have undoubtedly achieved the developmental task level of intimacy as described by Erik Erikson (1963). This becomes a difficult, if not impossible, task to achieve when there is an adolescent pregnancy.

A review of the dimensions of adaptation that have just been discussed shows that a variety of categories exist in which client data may be significant and from which nursing diagnoses may be formulated. Table 11-1 lists nursing diagnoses that have potential for use in the antepartal period. When viewing these diagnoses it is important to realize that they are very general and are made specific to the individual client when used in the context of the nursing process.

Table 11-1 Nursing Diagnoses with Potential for Use During the Antepartal Period

At risk for abnormal fetal development

Alterations in maternal nutrition

Alterations in maternal metabolism

Disruptions in the fetal-placental unit

Alterations in fetal physiological state

Alterations in hormonal and gastrointestinal functioning during the
  first trimester of pregnancy

Alterations in body mechanics

Ineffective family coping patterns

Alterations in patterns of sexuality

Alterations in body image

Alterations in role expectations

Client Situation

Kim was a 15 year old white female who presented at the neighborhood health clinic stating that she was pregnant. She was a high school sophomore who lived with her parents and four younger brothers and sisters. Although the family was in the middle income group, Kim's father had been on strike for eight weeks, and income had been limited.

Kim had many concerns about being pregnant. During the history she made the following statement: "I am ashamed and afraid my family and friends will reject me when they know I'm pregnant." The initial person Kim confided in regarding her pregnancy was her girlfriend, who convinced her to tell her parents. Kim told her mother about her suspicion that she was pregnant. Kim's mother made the appointment for the first prenatal visit. Kim's comment to the nurse was that her parents were very upset. She stated: "They told me I was a disgrace to the family." Kim related that she was afraid something was wrong with her: "I've been nauseated and vomiting all the time." Kim stuttered during the interview, her lower lip trembled, her eyes became watery, and her voice at times was low.

Dietary history revealed Kim ate a diet low in protein with an abundance of carbohydrates and empty calories. Kim stated that she liked milk and ate meat once a day. A 24-hour dietary recall of the previous day revealed two glasses of milk, two candy bars, one hamburger with cheese, french fries, three sodas and two doughnuts. Kim stated that her family rarely had meals together and family dietary habits were similar to hers.

Other data obtained through the assessment provided the following information:

History Past health history negative for significant disease. No cardio-vascular, renal, or endocrine disease. Family history revealed a maternal grandmother with diabetes and a father with hypertension.

Onset of menarche at age 13. Date of last menstrual period was 4/15; expected date of confinement 1/22. There had been no previous pregnancies.

Physical Examination B.P. 100/70, pulse 90, respiration 20. Ear, nose, throat, chest, breast, neurologic system, and extremities: negative findings. Abdomen: gravid. Bimanual pelvic exam revealed gynecoid pelvis of adequate size for 7 pound baby. Uterus: gravid — 14 week size.

Laboratory Data
Pregnancy test: positive
Urine: negative for glucose and protein
Blood type: O positive
Gonococcal culture and VDRL for syphilis: negative
Rubella titer: Reactive (Indicating immune response to rubella viremia)
Hemoglobin: 10.4 gm/100ml (Normal: 12 to 16 gm/100 ml)
Hematocrit: 31 per cent (Normal: 37 to 47 per cent)

With the data available to the nurse from assessment, combined with the knowledge and experience the nurse brought to this client situation, the nurse proceeded to sort the assessment data according to its significance for nursing diagnoses. Data which was highly significant was examined for patterns or clusters and these data items, grouped together, formed the bases for the nursing diagnoses.

The nursing diagnoses formulated from Kim's data are:

1. Threat to developmental tasks of adolescence associated with unwanted pregnancy.

2. Depressed support system related to socially unacceptable pregnancy.

3. Inadequate nutritional status associated with poor dietary habits.

4. Fear related to lack of knowledge of the normal accompaniments of pregnancy.

_____ **NURSING DIAGNOSIS** _____

Threat to developmental tasks of adolescence associated with unwanted pregnancy.

Assessment

Significant assessment data that formed the basis for this nursing diagnosis included:

1. Unwed adolescent who was 14 weeks pregnant.
2. Many signs of anxiety demonstrated during history and physical exam.
3. No prenatal care for first 3½ months of pregnancy.
4. Developmental crisis of adolescence superimposed on crisis of unwanted pregnancy.

Plan

The plan for this diagnosis is to promote Kim's development as an adolescent by enhancing her self-esteem and to support her independence.

Intervention

Nursing Interventions	Rationale	Outcome Criteria
1. Involve Kim in decision-making activities relative to the outcomes of pregnancy.	Participation in decision-making promotes an individual's sense of control.	Kim will take responsibility for her decisions and show signs of increasing maturity.
2. Praise Kim for her accomplishments as the pregnancy proceeds.	Positive reinforcement and praise help promote a positive sense of self.	Kim's self-concept will improve; she will begin to make positive statements about herself.
3. Encourage expression of feelings by Kim about herself and her pregnancy.	Reviewing feelings about self is part of the experience of pregnancy. The adolescent is often ashamed and uncomfortable with her pregnant body (Clark and Affonso, 1979)	Kim will begin to share some of her feelings with the nurse.
4. Be available for Kim during prenatal visits.	Communicating a sense of availability facilitates the development of trust, which is the initial step in any relationship.	Kim will talk with the nurse during prenatal visits with increasing ease and readiness.

_____ NURSING DIAGNOSIS _____

Depressed support system related to socially unacceptable pregnancy.

Assessment

Significant assessment data that formed the basis for this diagnosis included:

1. Kim's statement, "I am ashamed and afraid my family and friends will reject me when they know I'm pregnant."

2. Kim's appearance during the interview: She stuttered, her lower lip trembled, her eyes became watery, and her voice at times was low.

3. Kim's statement that her parents were critical of her for becoming pregnant.

4. The knowledge that anxiety is experienced when there is a threat to a biological need or threat to the security of the self (Clark and Affonso, 1979).

Plan

Promote the development of a support system between Kim and her family.

Intervention

Nursing Interventions	Rationale	Outcome Criteria
1. Allow time for ventilation of feelings.	Ventilation of feelings reduces mild anxiety and helps to reduce the feelings of threat to self (Clark and Affonso, 1979).	Kim will discuss feelings about her family and herself.
2. Encourage Kim to discuss with her parents her pregnancy, her prenatal care, and her economic and educational needs and concerns.	Positive communication promotes understanding and acceptance (Jensen and coworkers, 1977).	Tension between Kim and her parents will begin to decrease. Kim will make decisions about her future with support from her parents.

_____ NURSING DIAGNOSIS _____

Inadequate nutritional status associated with poor dietary habits.

Assessment

This nursing diagnosis was made on the basis of the following significant data:

1. History of low protein diet with an abundance of carbohydrates and empty calories.

2. Hemoglobin: 10.4 gm/100 ml.
   Hematocrit: 31 per cent.

3. Poor family dietary habits. The family rarely eats meals together.

4. Knowledge that Kim's diet is typical of many adolescents.

5. Knowledge that there is a correlation between fetal outcome and nutrition.

Plan

To increase Kim's intake of essential nutrients.

Intervention

Nursing Interventions	Rationale	Outcome Criteria
1. Review nutritional needs during pregnancy with client and her mother, since mother will prepare food at home.	Nutrition is significant in fetal outcome. The preparer of the food should be aware of the significance of the diet so that she will be motivated to alter foods presented for the family (Barnes, 1968).	Kim's mother will become aware of the relationship between nutrition and fetal outcome as demonstrated by an increase in nutritional foods prepared at home.
2. Review the basic four food groups and foods high in iron and folic acid. Encourage client to take prenatal vitamins.	It is necessary for the patient and her mother to know foods that contain appropriate nutrients (Williams, 1973).	Kim will increase her intake of protein and decrease the amount of empty calories she consumes. Intake of food containing iron will increase, and she will take her prenatal vitamins.
3. Refer patient to WIC (Women, Infant and Children) program. (This is a federal program to improve the outcome of pregnancy by improving maternal nutrition).	Kim's pregnancy is at risk because of her age, 15, her poor dietary habits, and the family's financial distress, which affects their food-purchasing ability. The outcome of pregnancy can be improved by providing proper nutrients for those patients at highest risk (United States Department of Agriculture, Food and Nutritional Service, 1978).	Kim's mother will obtain and utilize WIC vouchers to purchase foods that Kim needs during her pregnancy.

Nursing Interventions (Cont'd)	*Rationale (Cont'd)*	*Outcome Criteria (Cont'd)*
4. Instruct patient in foods that are economical and high in protein, iron, and folic acid.	If the client has a knowledge of foods high in nutrients and low in cost, this will increase the likelihood of her ability to purchase food of higher nutritional value (Williams, 1973).	Hemoglobin and hematocrit levels will increase.

NURSING DIAGNOSIS

Fear related to lack of knowledge of the normal accompaniments of pregnancy.

Assessment

Significant data that formed the basis for this nursing diagnosis were:

1. Kim's statement that she was "afraid something was wrong with her."
2. Kim's complaint of frequent nausea and vomiting.
3. The knowledge that pregnant women experience nausea and vomiting during the first trimester of pregnancy.

Plan

To reduce Kim's fear and alleviate the severity of her symptoms.

Intervention

Nursing Interventions	*Rationale*	*Outcome Criteria*
1. Reassure Kim that her nausea and vomiting are normal symptoms of pregnancy.	Client needs to understand reason for experiencing nausea and vomiting so she does not fear something is wrong with her (Clausen and coworkers, 1976).	Kim will understand the cause of her nausea and vomiting and acknowledge them as normal manifestations of early pregnancy.
2. Teach Kim measures to reduce nausea and vomiting. a. Avoid situations that produce nausea; for example, if a certain odor makes her nauseous, she should avoid it.	If client knows methods of relieving nausea and vomiting, she will be able to cope with the symptoms. (Clausen and coworkers, 1976).	Kim will utilize measures to reduce the amount of nausea and vomiting.

Nursing Interventions (Cont'd)　　　*Rationale (Cont'd)*　　　*Outcome Criteria (Cont'd)*

   b. Reassure Kim that
      nausea and vomiting
      usually dissipate after
      the first trimester.
   c. Encourage Kim to rise
      slowly in the morning
      and to eat a soda
      cracker or a dry piece
      of toast before getting
      out of bed.
   d. Encourage the avoid-
      ance of greasy foods.
   e. Encourage measures to
      reduce emotional
      tensions.

Evaluation Summary

Kim was able to adjust to the many demands that her pregnancy placed upon her. She attended each scheduled prenatal visit and preparation for childbirth class. By the second clinic visit, Kim had greatly improved her nutritional status by increasing her protein intake 25 grams per day. Kim's mother had obtained food vouchers from the social worker to purchase additional eggs, juice, and other foods high in protein and vitamin content. Kim's hemoglobin had increased to 11 gm/100 ml, and her hematocrit level was 33 per cent.

Relationships between Kim and the other family members improved. She stated that parents and siblings were spending more time with her. She attended a school for pregnant teenagers and received much support from this group. Kim's goals for further education after the baby's birth had already been developed.

Kim decided to place her baby for adoption. There had been an agreement with an organization for family and children's services to place the baby for adoption. Special attention was provided for Kim by the social worker to assist her in working through the grief of relinquishing her baby. With the support of her family and health care providers, Kim developed a more positive sense of self.

THE INTRAPARTAL PERIOD

The second model that will be presented encompasses caring for a patient during her labor and delivery experience. There are unique assessment parameters that are applied to the intrapartal period because of the nature of labor and delivery. Nursing care during the intrapartal period should be individualized to meet the mother's needs and to make the birth of the baby a memorable and pleasant event. To provide this type of nursing care, the nurse must be well skilled in nursing assessment, in establishing nursing diagnoses, and in supportive techniques during labor to help promote comfort. The father should be given high priority, and if he has elected to coach his wife, the nurse has the job of helping him to feel comfortable and effective in his participation (Clark and Affonso, 1979).

The birth of the baby is a very significant event in the family, and the nurse has the opportunity to provide comfort and to help assure a positive and healthy outcome for both mother and baby. The mother has much anticipation during her pregnancy about what the labor experience will be like, and as her pregnancy draws to a close, she will want to know when she should go to the hospital and when she is in true labor. It is also very important that the nurse know signs of true and false labor to effectively evaluate the patient's labor. The data in Table 11–2 is used for evaluating true and false labor.

Table 11–2   Indications of True and False Labor*

Parameter	True Labor	False Labor
Contractions	Regular	Irregular
Intervals between contractions	Gradually shorten	No change
Duration and severity of contractions	Increase	No change
Location of pain	Starts in back and moves to front	Mainly in front
Intensity of pain	Increases with walking	No change with walking
Association between degree of uterine hardening and intensity of pain	Present	No relationship
Bloody show	Often present	No show
Cervix	Becomes effaced and dilated	No change
Presenting part	Descent	No descent
Head	Fixed between pains	Head remains full
Sedation	No effect on true labor	Will stop false labor

*Adapted from Oxorn and Foote, 1968

After the decision has been made that the patient is in true labor, the nurse continues to assess the patient. The baby's heart rate is checked with a fetalscope every 15 minutes when the patient is in active labor to assure the well-being of the baby. The normal range for the fetal heart rate is 120 to 160 beats per minute. The nurse also checks the mother's vital signs every

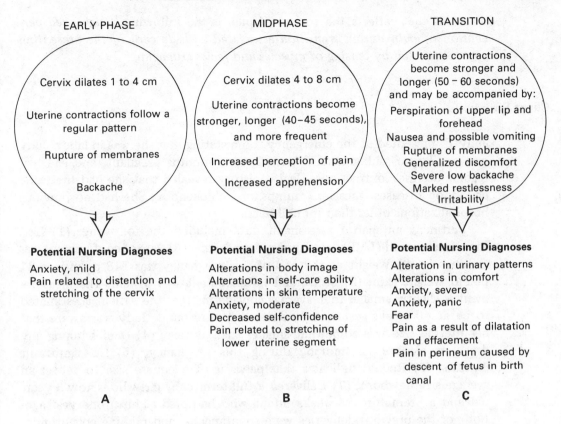

EARLY PHASE

Cervix dilates 1 to 4 cm

Uterine contractions follow a regular pattern

Rupture of membranes

Backache

Potential Nursing Diagnoses

Anxiety, mild
Pain related to distention and stretching of the cervix

A

MIDPHASE

Cervix dilates 4 to 8 cm

Uterine contractions become stronger, longer (40–45 seconds), and more frequent

Increased perception of pain

Increased apprehension

Potential Nursing Diagnoses

Alterations in body image
Alterations in self-care ability
Alterations in skin temperature
Anxiety, moderate
Decreased self-confidence
Pain related to stretching of lower uterine segment

B

TRANSITION

Uterine contractions become stronger and longer (50 – 60 seconds) and may be accompanied by:
Perspiration of upper lip and forehead
Nausea and possible vomiting
Rupture of membranes
Generalized discomfort
Severe low backache
Marked restlessness
Irritability

Potential Nursing Diagnoses

Alteration in urinary patterns
Alterations in comfort
Anxiety, severe
Anxiety, panic
Fear
Pain as a result of dilatation and effacement
Pain in perineum caused by descent of fetus in birth canal

C

Figure 11-2 Potential nursing diagnoses for the intrapartal period.

hour to rule out the development of any complications. The patient's labor pattern is evaluated for progress of effacement and dilatation. Effacement is the thinning of the cervix; dilatation is the opening of the cervix (the range is 0 to 10 cm) (Jensen and coworkers, 1977).

Labor can be divided into three main phases: early, midphase, and transition. Wiedenbach (1967) has developed a "stages of labor" chart, which is a guide for supporting mothers during labor. Components of each phase provide a basis for the listing of potential nursing diagnoses for the intrapartal period (Figure 11–2 A, B, and C).

In this model, nursing diagnoses utilizing the framework of adaptation will be developed. The laboring patient makes many adaptations, most of which are directed at relieving discomfort and anxiety so that she will be able to participate optimally in the birth of her child.

Maternal physiological adaptation needs to be carefully assessed during labor, particularly the response to pain and discomfort. The source of the pain, which varies with the stage of labor, needs to be indicated when the assessment and nursing diagnoses are made. Laboratory and clinical studies suggest that pain during the first stage of labor is primarily caused by the dilatation of the cervix with distention, stretching, and possible tearing of this structure (Clark and Affonso, 1979). Pain during transition and the second stage of labor is produced primarily by distention of the lower birth canal and perineum (Clark and Affonso, 1979). An example of a nursing diagnosis that reflects the source of pain is the following: *heightened perception of pain during transition associated with descent of the presenting part manifested by tensing of muscles and facial grimacing.*

Client Situation

Judy B. presented at the emergency room stating that she was in labor. Judy was a 27 year old gravida 3 para 2, nine months pregnant, and she had regular uterine contractions. Health history revealed that she had the usual childhood diseases: measles, mumps, and chickenpox. She had no previous hospitalizations other than for childbirth.

Pertinent antepartal assessment data included the following: (1) Last menstrual period (LMP) was January 1, and expected date of confinement was October 8; (2) Weight at the end of this pregnancy was 148 pounds, a 31 pound weight gain; (3) McDonald measurement was 31 cm. The measurement is slightly smaller than average considering that the patient is estimated to be at 40 weeks gestation by dates and ultrasound. Judy was aware that her uterine size was somewhat smaller than average; (4) Denies taking any drugs or alcohol or smoking during this pregnancy; (5) No significant illnesses; (6) Record indicates that pelvis is of adequate size to deliver an average size newborn; (7) Delivered a full-term baby girl who is now 3 years old and a premature 24-weeks infant who had died at birth one year ago. Both of the previous deliveries were spontaneous, and midline episiotomies were performed.

Further assessment revealed that Judy was anxious; she was holding tightly to her husband's hand and was talking in a low modulated voice. She had glassy almost tearful eyes when she reported, "I'm in labor and my membranes have ruptured." The vital signs were as follows: temperature 98.6, pulse 96, respirations 20. Judy was having contractions that started in the back and radiated to the lower abdomen, occurring every five minutes. Judy stated that she was having a moderate amount of discomfort with the contractions. The nurse assessed Judy's adaptation to the contractions and found that she was attempting to use the breathing techniques taught in her Lamaze childbirth class, but she was hyperventilating. The nurse assessed for rupture of membranes through the use of the nitrazine and fern tests, both of which indicated the presence of amniotic fluid; Judy's membranes had ruptured.

To this point, data gathered from Mrs. B. clustered in categories that formed the bases for the nursing diagnostic statements. The discomforts of the uterine contractions, the ruptured membranes, and misuse of breathing techniques leading to hyperventilation suggested that this was a patient in early labor who could benefit from nursing intervention so that she would feel in control and relaxed with her labor.

The nursing diagnoses made for Judy included:

1. Alterations in comfort associated with uterine contractions of early labor.

2. Anxiety about the birth of baby associated with past experience of death of premature infant.

3. Risk for the development of chorioamnionitis related to premature rupture of membranes.

4. Risk for prolapse of umbilical cord associated with fetal head being at a minus station and premature rupture of the membranes.

5. Increased perception of pain related to dilatation of the cervix and contractions of the midphase of labor.

6. At risk for compromised uterine blood supply associated with strong uterine contractions.

7. Increased apprehension and heightened perception of pain associated with the stretching of the lower uterine segment during transition and birth.

The first two nursing diagnoses are directed toward meeting the patient's needs during early labor. Wiedenbach (1967) has described patients' behavior during early labor as one of anticipation, relief, and some apprehension. Judy's behavior in labor was compounded by the loss of her second infant. She was very concerned about the health and well-being of this baby and needed reassurances about the baby's condition during labor.

_____ NURSING DIAGNOSIS _____

Alterations in comfort associated with uterine contractions of early labor.

Assessment

Data significant for the formulation of this nursing diagnosis included:

1. No history of antepartal complications.

2. Presence of regular uterine contractions starting in the back and radiating to the lower abdomen.

3. Membranes ruptured as indicated by positive nitrazine and fern tests.

4. Judy is 40 weeks gestation by dates, but her McDonald measurement is somewhat small for the number of weeks of gestation. She is concerned that the baby is small because the doctor said her uterus is small for date.

5. Judy has attended childbirth classes and desires to use breathing techniques to work through her labor contractions.

Plan

In this situation the nursing plan includes efforts to decrease the discomforts of early labor by assisting the patient in breathing, relaxation, and supportive techniques.

Intervention

Nursing Interventions*	Rationale	Outcome Criteria
1. Orient Mr. and Mrs. B. to labor room.	This helps the couple feel more comfortable and at ease in their surroundings.	Mr. and Mrs. B. will feel comfortable and relaxed in labor room environment.
2. Review breathing techniques for labor with Judy.	Use of appropriate breathing techniques helps the patient cope with the discomforts of contractions.	Judy will demonstrate appropriate breathing techniques.
3. Review relaxation techniques with Judy.	If the patient is able to relax, it will help reduce perception of pain. Relaxation enables the woman to obtain maximum benefit from the rest periods between contractions to reduce fatigue and increase her energy. This allows her to return to the task of labor refreshed and revitalized (Clark and Affonso, 1979).	Judy will relax extremities. She will be in control of her breathing and be able to cope with the discomforts of labor.
4. Teach Judy signs of hyperventilation, that is, tingling hands and feelings of dizziness.	Patients often hyperventilate during labor because of rapid breathing patterns, and this results in the loss of CO_2. Being informed about signs of hyperventilation may prevent its occurrence.	Judy will recognize signs of hyperventilation and will be able to verbalize these signs.
5. Teach interventions to counteract hyperventilation: a. Slow down rate of breathing. b. Hold breath for short time.	If patient knows methods of counteracting hyperventilation, she will be able to use slow, deep breathing, which will conserve CO_2.	Judy will be able to counteract effects of hyperventilation.
6. Support husband in his role as coach.	The nurse has the responsibility to help other persons give support to the mother during labor. If the husband feels comfortable in his role, he will be a more effective coach to his wife (Clark and Affonso, 1979).	Mr. B. will coach his wife in labor. His assistance will promote Judy's comfort.

*Editor's note: Interventions listed in this intrapartal model incorporate the ongoing nursing assessments made throughout the stages of labor. Assessment is included here to convey the scope of nursing actions with the intrapartal patient.

Nursing Interventions (Cont'd)	Rationale (Cont'd)	Outcome Criteria (Cont'd)
7. Reassure Judy regarding her baby's condition. Check fetal heart rate every 15 minutes and let Judy listen to the baby's heart beat.	If the mother is assured of the well-being of the baby, her anxiety will be allayed.	Judy will be informed of the baby's status and reassured that the fetal heart tones are normal.
8. Time contractions and evaluate contractions for duration and intensity.	It is important to know the status of the contractions; for labor to progress contractions usually last 45 to 60 seconds. A contraction lasting longer than 90 seconds could lead to fetal hypoxia. It is important that the uterine muscle relax between contractions to promote optimal exchange of oxygen via the fetal-placental unit (Pritchard and McDonald, 1976).	Contractions will get closer together as labor progresses, and contractions will last at least 45 seconds and be of moderate intensity without signs of uterine dysfunction.
9. Check cervical dilatation, station, and effacement by sterile vaginal exam when indicated by signs of progress of labor.	The need for sterile vaginal exams to check cervical dilatation depends on the progress of labor. Usually hourly or bi-hourly examinations are sufficient to determine if the pattern of cervical dilatation is within normal limits when plotted on the Friedman Curve (Friedman, 1978).	Patient's dilatation will increase approximately 1 cm per hour, the fetal head will progress to a lower station, and effacement will be 100 per cent.

Evaluation

Judy was able to maintain control of her breathing and relax between contractions. The contractions came at regular intervals, and the interval between contractions shortened from 5 minutes to 3 minutes. At 0900, Judy's cervical dilatation was 3 cm, 60 per cent effaced, and –1 station. Her contractions had become stronger, and she was also having more difficulty controlling her response to pain. The fetal heart tones had remained between 130 and 140 beats/minute. The progress of Judy's labor at this time was within normal limits.

_____ NURSING DIAGNOSIS _____

Anxiety about the birth of baby associated with past experience of death of premature infant.

The second nursing diagnosis is related to Judy's anxiety about her baby's condition. This anxiety stems from the previous loss of a preterm infant. Judy related further that she had not prepared at home for the baby because she was afraid of another disappointment. She has not demonstrated nesting behavior, that is, the behavior demonstrated by the mother during pregnancy in which she gathers together clothing, the baby bed, and other materials she will need for baby care (Rubin, 1970). Absence of nesting behavior can sometimes suggest a potential for a lag in bonding behaviors between mother and baby (Klaus and Kennell, 1976).

Assessment

Data significant to the formulation of this diagnosis included:

1. Husband is supportive of wife.

2. Patient relates that she is anxious about this baby's condition. She is afraid something will be wrong with the baby.

3. She continually wrings her hands and asks many questions about the well-being of the baby.

4. Previous infant died at birth. The infant was premature (24 weeks gestation).

5. Patient has not demonstrated nesting behaviors.

6. Patient is concerned that her uterine size is small and is afraid this means she has a small baby.

7. The fetal heart tones are within normal limits.

Plan

The nursing plan is to reduce Judy's anxiety about the condition of the baby.

Intervention

Nursing Interventions	Rationale	Outcome Criteria
1. Allow time for Judy to verbalize her concerns and fears.	Verbalizing concerns can help reduce anxiety and bring fears into a more rational perspective.	Judy will verbalize concerns and show a reduction in signs of anxiety.

Nursing Interventions (Cont'd)	*Rationale (Cont'd)*	*Outcome Criteria (Cont'd)*
2. When listening to the fetal heart rate, allow Judy to listen.	Listening to the baby's heart beat assures the mother of the baby's well-being.	Judy will state she is less anxious.
3. Reassure Judy that she is 40 weeks gestation and her labor is progressing without complications.	Judy's fear is related to the birth of a previous premature infant. She needs reassurance that this baby is fully developed and is being born in a completely different set of circumstances.	Judy can acknowledge that her labor is progressing normally.

Evaluation

Judy seemed to be reassured of her baby's well-being after listening to the fetal heart tones. As labor progressed, the nurse established a positive rapport with the patient, and the patient became less anxious.

The third and fourth nursing diagnoses deal with the premature rupture of membranes, a condition that increases the risk for the development of chorioamnionitis. If the membranes have been ruptured for longer than 24 hours, the morbidity from chorioamnionitis increases for mother and baby. If the baby's head is not engaged and the membranes are ruptured, the umbilical cord may slip down or prolapse between the presenting part and the cervix or other part of the birth canal. A prolapse of the cord makes the cord more susceptible to being compressed, thereby decreasing the blood flow and oxygenation of the fetus (Danforth, 1977).

_____ NURSING DIAGNOSIS _____

Risk for the development of chorioamnionitis related to premature rupture of membranes.

Assessment Data

Significant data for this nursing diagnosis included:

1. Membranes ruptured spontaneously as confirmed by positive nitrazine and fern tests.

2. Membranes ruptured at 0200 hours, 7 hours ago.

3. No signs of variable deceleration of the fetal heart beat, which would be a sign of cord compression.

4. Doctor ordered bedrest for Judy to prevent prolapse of the cord.

Plan

For this situation, the nurse's plan is to prevent the development of chorioamnionitis.

Intervention

Nursing Interventions	Rationale	Outcome Criteria
1. Perform vaginal examinations with appropriate aseptic precautions and only as frequently as is absolutely necessary.	Vaginal exams more frequent than necessary may increase the risk of infection being introduced.	Vaginal exams will be performed only when needed, thereby decreasing risk of introduction of infection.

_____ NURSING DIAGNOSIS _____

Risk for prolapse of umbilical cord associated with fetal head being at a minus station and premature rupture of the membranes.

Assessment

Significant data for this nursing diagnosis included:

1. Spontaneous rupture of membranes.
2. Fetal head at minus station.

Plan

The nursing plan is to prevent prolapse of the umbilical cord.

Intervention

Nursing Interventions	Rationale	Outcome Criteria
1. Place patient in recumbent position to prevent prolapse of the cord. Explain to patient the reason for this restriction of position.	If the patient remains recumbent, this will safeguard against prolapse of the cord (Jensen and coworkers, 1977).	Patient will remain in recumbent position during labor and understands the need for this position.

Nursing Interventions (Cont'd)	*Rationale (Cont'd)*	*Outcome Criteria (Cont'd)*
2. Periodic fetal heart rate monitoring to determine fetal well-being.	Fetal heart rate should be checked regularly during labor in order to help recognize any complications that may develop in the baby. Cord compression causes variable decelerations in the monitor strip if the patient is being monitored (Hon, 1975).	Fetal heart rate within normal limits (120 to 160).
3. Observe for passage of meconium, a possible sign of fetal distress with a vertex presentation.	It is necessary to watch for signs of fetal distress in order to recognize deviations in the fetal condition that need immediate intervention.	No passage of meconium will be found.
4. Inspect for presence of cord when performing vaginal examination.	The potential exists for the cord to prolapse when the head is not engaged and the membranes are ruptured.	No cord found on vaginal examination. Physician notified immediately if prolapse is detected.

Evaluation

At 1000 Judy's contractions were 3 minutes apart, 45 seconds long, and strong in intensity. Judy stated that she didn't know if she'd be able to keep up with this breathing. The nurse encouraged her to continue, stating, "You're doing a great job and making progress." At this time the nurse performed a sterile vaginal examination and found Judy to be 5 cm dilated and 100 per cent effaced at 0 station. The nurse informed the patient of her progress; Judy was very pleased and continued to work with the breathing and relaxation exercises. The nurse checked fetal heart tones and found them to be 130 with a regular beat-to-beat variability.

The patient is now in the midphase of her labor. Wiedenbach (1967) states that the patient may feel apprehensive. She may feel a growing sense of ill-defined doubts and fears. She has a desire for companionship, and she may feel uncertain about whether she can cope with contractions.

_____ NURSING DIAGNOSIS _____

Increased perception of pain related to dilatation of the cervix and contractions of the mid-phase of labor.

Assessment

Data significant to the formulation of this diagnosis included:

1. Contractions intense, lasting 45 seconds, and 3 minutes apart.
2. Judy's statement, "I don't know if I can do this breathing much longer."
3. Sterile vaginal exam reveals 5 cm dilatation; 100 per cent effaced, 0 station.
4. Signs of fetal distress not present. Fetal heart rate within normal limits. Amniotic fluid clear; no meconium staining.

Plan

The nurse's plan is to promote Judy's sense of control in her progress through labor.

Intervention

Nursing Interventions	Rationale	Outcome Criteria
1. Use comfort measures to reduce perception of pain: a. Encourage voluntary muscle release. b. Apply counter pressure to sacrococcygeal area. c. Utilize effleurage (gentle stroking of the abdomen), if patient desires. d. Cool cloth to forehead. e. Give mouth care.	Comfort measures help patient to relax and to cope with labor more effectively.	Patient seems more relaxed and able to cope with pain after comfort measures are applied.
2. Encourage and praise patient.	Positive reinforcement promotes continuation of learned breathing and relaxation techniques, and praise enhances self-esteem.	With positive reinforcement, patient maintains control, and self-esteem is enhanced.
3. Encourage patient to void to relieve pressure of full bladder and prevent bladder distention.	A full bladder is uncomfortable and impedes the progress of labor.	Bladder is not distended.

Evaluation

Judy responded well to encouragement and support during the midphase of her labor. She was able to concentrate on her breathing exercises; no hyperventilation was noted. She responded happily to information that she was making progess in her labor.

_____ NURSING DIAGNOSIS _____

At risk for compromised uterine blood supply associated with strong uterine contractions.

Assessment

Significant data for this nursing diagnosis included:

1. Contractions lasting 45 seconds, 3 minutes apart.
2. Patient lying in supine position.

Plan

The nursing plan for this diagnosis is to maximize the available blood supply to the fetus.

Intervention

Nursing Interventions	Rationale	Outcome Criteria
1. Position patient on left side to reduce pressure on the vena cava and increase blood flow to the uterus	The pressure of the gravid uterus on the vena cava can compromise the blood flow to the uterus. Positioning the patient on her left side improves blood flow to the uterus by reducing pressure on the vena cava (Pritchard and McDonald, 1976).	Vena cava syndrome not present; maternal blood pressure will remain within normal limits. Fetal heart rate will remain within normal limits.
2. Observe for signs of fetal distress by checking fetal heart rate and heart monitor readout for variable decelerations and decreasing beat-to-beat variability.	Alterations in fetal heart rate are a reliable indicator of fetal distress (Hon, 1975).	No sign of fetal distress.

Evaluation

At 1100 Judy was having more difficulty controlling breathing, and she showed marked restlessness. She told the nurse, "I can't take it. I can't stand this any longer. Can't you do something?" Judy's behavior demonstrates signs of transition. The nurse does a sterile vaginal examination, which reveals the following: 8 cm dilatation, 100 per cent effaced, and +1 station. The fetal heart tones are 140. The nurse also observes the patient has beads of perspiration on her forehead and above her lip. Wiedenbach (1967) correlates these symptoms with transition. The nurse tells the patient she is having the longest and strongest contractions that she will have until she is completely dilated. At 11:30 Judy is completely dilated and begins to push with each contraction.

_____ **NURSING DIAGNOSIS** _____

Increased apprehension and heightened perception of pain associated with the stretching of the lower uterine segment during transition and birth.

Assessment

Data significant to the formulation of this nursing diagnosis included:

1. Signs of restlessness and increased perspiration.
2. Difficulty controlling rhythmic breathing.
3. Statements suggesting a perceived loss of control.
4. Cervix dilated to 8 cm with 100 per cent effacement.

Plan

The nurse will promote comfort and support during transition and delivery.

Intervention

Nursing Interventions	Rationale	Outcome Criteria
1. Reassure both patient and spouse that labor is progressing normally.	Knowledge that labor is progressing normally reduces patient's fears.	Patient and spouse will acknowledge that labor is proceeding normally.
2. Encourage both patient and spouse to use psychophysical breathing techniques appropriate for transition.	Active coaching of the labor patient for the phase of transition helps patient maintain control (Clark and Affonso, 1979).	Patient utilizes breathing techniques appropriate for transition.

Nursing Interventions (Cont'd)	Rationale (Cont'd)	Outcome Criteria (Cont'd)
3. Keep patient informed of progress of labor and status of baby.	If patient understands she is making progress, this helps her to cope with the discomforts of transition.	Patient recognizes she is making progress in her labor and that her baby's fetal heart tones are normal.
4. Instruct patient to push when she reaches 10 cm dilatation.	Pushing when completely dilated facilitates the birth of the baby during the second stage of labor.	Baby descends in birth canal when mother is pushing.
5. Accompany patient to delivery room. Explain procedures and techniques as they occur in order to relieve pain and apprehension.	Explanation of procedures by a consistent coach helps the patient maintain control of her labor.	Pain and apprehension relieved.
6. As baby is delivering, allow husband to stay with his wife and encourage him to participate as much as possible in the birth of their baby.	The husband is significant in offering comfort to his wife. People who witness the birth process become strongly attached to the infant (Kennell and Rolnick, 1960).	Husband coaches his wife in the delivery room and will be present for the birth of their baby.
7. Allow parents to hold the baby and maintain eye contact with baby in delivery room.	The time immediately after the birth of the baby is considered to be a sensitive time for bonding to take place. If the parents desire to hold their baby, they should be afforded this opportunity (Klaus and Kennell, 1976).	Parents will hold and maintain eye contact if they desire to do so.
8. Examine baby as soon as possible and allow couple to observe examination.	Knowledge that the baby is normal and adapting to her new environment relieves the parent's anxiety.	Patient and spouse are reassured that their baby is normal.

Evaluation

Judy gave birth to a 5 pound, 7 ounce baby girl. The baby's physical examination was within normal limits except the baby was small for gestational age. The baby had a normal course in the nursery. The pregnancy, labor, and delivery were without complications, and the family is adapting well to the birth of their baby.

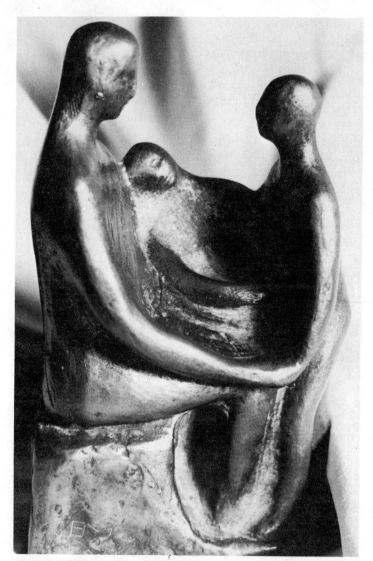

THE POSTPARTAL PERIOD

The postpartal period is the time from the birth of the baby until the uterus returns to its normal pre-pregnant state. During this period there are many rapid physiological and psychological adaptations for the new mother. The mother's responses to the adaptive demands provide the data base for the formulation of nursing diagnoses specific to the postpartal period.

Physiological Dimension

There are many maternal physiological adjustments after the birth of the baby, all of which require thorough assessment by the nurse.

The vital signs are very important to assess in the postpartal period to detect the development of complications. A fall in blood pressure and an increase in pulse rate may suggest a postpartal hemorrhage; other changes in the vital signs may point to other complications.

Involution of the uterus to its pre-pregnant state is an important physiological adaptation to assess. Immediately after delivery, the uterus should be contracted, firm, and approximately one finger-breadth below the umbilicus. Each postpartal day thereafter, the uterus should involute approximately one finger breadth below the umbilicus until involution is complete. The nurse palpates the uterus to determine if it is firm, midline, and involuting properly.

Alterations in uterine involution is a nursing diagnosis that is seen with some degree of frequency on the postpartal unit. Such alterations usually indicate a boggy uterus and may be related to a lack of uterine tone, infection, fibroids, retained placental fragments, or a distended bladder.

The type of lochia is also assessed on a daily basis for its color, consistency, amount, and odor. The lochia is the vaginal flow after delivery composed of the necrotic superficial layer of the myometrium and blood from the uterine sinuses at the placental site (Clark and Affonso, 1979). The lochia during the first 3 days is bright red and is known as lochia rubra. The lochia then changes to pink or brown (3 to 8 days) and is known as lochia serosa. By the tenth day the lochia turns creamy white and is called lochia alba. Alterations in lochia, such as a profuse amount with large clots, constitute the basis for a nursing diagnosis and may be related to a hemorrhage or laceration.

Healing of the episiotomy is also assessed by the nurse. If the episiotomy is healing properly, the incision will be intact with possible swelling caused by the trauma of birth; there should be no excessive signs of inflammation, that is, redness, purulent discharge, or foul odor. Discomfort from the episiotomy is also important to assess. If discomfort is present, an analgesic may be given along with routine sitz baths to promote comfort and healing of the episiotomy site. Alterations in healing of the episiotomy provide a basis for nursing diagnoses in the immediate postpartal period.

The breasts of the mother have undergone physiological changes during pregnancy and the postpartal period and need to be assessed by the nurse. Through gentle palpation of each breast, the nurse assesses for engorgement, that is, firmness, tenderness, venous distention, and shiny breasts. A nursing diagnosis of excessive breast engorgement demands prompt intervention by the nurse to alleviate or prevent discomfort. The nurse assesses the let-down reflex, the release of milk caused by a neuro-hormonal reflex that is stimulated by the baby's suckling. Also assessed are the nipples to determine if there are any cracks or fissures that could lead to sore nipples and possible breast infection. Alterations in nipple status yield additional diagnoses.

Bowel and bladder functions are other important physiological parameters to assess in the postpartal period. After delivery the nurse may detect that the patient has a distended bladder. This may lead to excessive loss of blood because the bladder displaces the uterus and impedes the process of normal involution. The nurse must be aware that frequent small voidings or pain during urination may be signs of bladder infection. Alteration in bowel function, particularly constipation, is a common nursing diagnosis in the early postpartal period, and nursing intervention should be prompt.

Psychological Dimension

Reva Rubin (1961) has described two phases of psychological adaptation to motherhood, the taking-in phase and the taking-hold phase. The taking-in phase is characterized by dependency on the part of the mother. During this phase she is interested in sleep, food, reviewing the birth process, and beginning the claiming process of her baby. This is a time of regeneration for the mother, usually lasting two to three days. It is important to realize that the patient is a receiver at this time. Rubin (1961) states, "She accepts what she is given, tries to do what she is told, awaits the actions of others, and initiates very little herself."

The taking-hold phase ushers in the assertion of independence. During this phase the mother becomes the initiator; she wishes to take command of her life and is very interested in gaining skills to care for her baby. Rubin suggests that this phase is laden with anxiety for the mother and that mood swings are often seen during this period.

Alterations in progression through these phases serve as data for the formulation of nursing diagnoses.

Identity, self-concept, and mood are other important parameters to assess on the postpartal unit. If the mother has a strong sense of identity, she will be able to deal with the stresses of assuming a new role and the alterations in life style that a new baby causes. A positive self-concept in mother and father is a facilitating factor when the parents are adjusting to their new role. Body image is a part of the self-concept. Many mothers are distraught to find that their figures have not returned to the pre-pregnancy state (Iffrig, 1972). It is not an unusual sight on the postpartum unit to see a mother pat her abdomen and remark about the change, while some mothers look at their abdomens and shake their heads in dismay.

The mother's affect must also be assessed by the nurse. Fluctuations in mood may sometimes be seen on the postpartal unit. One such fluctuation is a temporary depression, commonly called "postpartum blues." This depression, characterized by crying and a "let down" feeling, is thought to be related to hormonal changes that occur at this time (Reeder and coworkers, 1976). The mother may find it particularly depressing to be unable to control her emotions (Clark and Affonso, 1979).

Social Dimension

Assessment of social parameters is very important because they affect the way individuals take on roles in society. Of particular interest is the taking on of the maternal role. Loss of self-definition in social roles is a problem that sometimes occurs in early motherhood (Clark and Affonso, 1979). Some mothers have difficulty adjusting to the loss of independence and the change in life style that a new baby brings. This can be particularly difficult if the mother has enjoyed a satisfying career (Clark and Affonso, 1979).

It is particularly important for the nurse to assess the development of the maternal-infant bond. This bond between mother and infant is considered to be a unique attachment, which endures through time and is crucial for the survival and development of the new infant (Klaus and Kennell, 1976). The strength of this bond makes it possible for the mother to sacrifice her own needs for those of her baby (Clark and Affonso, 1979). In assessing the progress of the mother-infant attachment it is important to consider that there is a "sensitive period" for the maternal-infant bonding that occurs in the early minutes and hours after birth. The nurse assesses the mother's reaction to her newborn and her subsequent reaction to her baby on the postpartal unit. Some mothers state that they feel more strongly attached to their baby after some time has elapsed. Alterations in maternal-infant bonding may lead to the development of nursing diagnoses on the postpartal unit.

Developmental Dimension

Assessment of the developmental level of the new mother is important. One very significant developmental milestone to be achieved by the new mother is the "taking on" of the maternal role. Many of her activities in the early postpartal period foster this role assumption and need to be assessed for their adequancy. For example, the new mother may repeatedly discuss her birth experience; such a review helps the mother incorporate and integrate this experience into an emerging behavior pattern consistent with the mothering role. Observations of the mother's growing competence and confidence in caring for her infant provides additional data about how adequately the mother is adapting to her new role.

The developmental tasks of the childbearing family should also be assessed. When a new member is added to the family, there is a forced reorganization of the roles and responsibilities of each of the members (Clark and Affonso, 1979). It is the developmental task of the family to make adjustments to accommodate the newest member.

Cultural Dimension

Cultural parameters affect the new mother's adaptation on the postpartal unit. After delivery, a woman and her family may exhibit behaviors that appear to conflict with those of the nurses' and physicians' concept of good postpartal care (Clark and Affonso, 1979). This may be due to cultural variations. Clark and Affonso (1979) suggest assessment of the following areas for cultural adaptation in the postpartal period: dietary intake, norms regarding maternal activities, precautions prescribed to protect the mother, and the type of support that is acceptable to her. Other important areas to assess are the influence of culture on parenting behaviors. Cultural variations that appear to hinder the mother's adaptation become the diagnoses that require nursing intervention.

In review, assessment by the nurse of the adaptive dimensions yields a number of potential nursing diagnoses appropriate to the postpartal period

(Table 11–3). Some of these diagnoses will be defined more specifically and used in the following client example.

Table 11–3 Potential Nursing Diagnoses for the Postpartal Period

Excessive lochia flow
Alterations in uterine involution
At risk for postpartal infection
At risk for breast engorgement
Inadequate milk supply in the breast-feeding mother
At risk for mastitis in the breast-feeding mother
Anxiety related to breast-feeding
Alterations of bowel and bladder function
Alterations in self-concept
Failure to assert independence, initiate self care, and assume the maternal role
Lag in maternal-infant bonding
Alteration in social roles
Lack of knowledge of child care
Difficulty adjusting to body image
Emotional lability associated with adaptation to parturition
At risk for postpartum psychosis

Client Situation

Mrs. G. has just given birth to her first child. She has been married for three years, during which time she has been employed as a grade school teacher. Her husband holds a management position with a Chicago firm. The couple resides in a suburb of Chicago where they have just purchased their first home. Mrs. G. has resigned her teaching position to stay home with the baby.

Mrs. G. slept soundly the first four hours after delivery. On waking, her first question was, "Can I see my baby?" The nurse responded that she would be bringing the infant in for rooming-in at 0900. Mrs. G. stated that she was disappointed with her labor and delivery because she had required general anesthesia. She and her husband had attended preparation for childbirth classes and had planned on being together for the delivery.

Mrs. G. also expressed concern about not feeding the baby since birth and asked the nurse if there would be someone to help her breast-feed. Mrs. G. then began to relate the details of her labor and delivery. She felt she was a failure, since she was not awake for delivery. Mrs. G. repeated several times, "I was a failure in delivery."

The nursing diagnoses for Mrs. G. are:

1. Alterations in self-concept associated with rigid expectations of the childbirth experience.

2. Alterations in uterine involution associated with decreased uterine tone.

3. Fear of breast-feeding related to a lack of knowledge and experience with breast-feeding.

4. Altered self-definition in social roles associated with changed life style following birth of baby.

5. Lack of knowledge and skill in baby care associated with child care inexperience.

_____ **NURSING DIAGNOSIS** _____

Alterations in self-concept associated with rigid expectations of the childbirth experience.

Assessment

Significant data for this first nursing diagnosis included:

1. Mrs. G. is in the taking-in phase.

2. Mrs. G.'s expectations of her labor experience were not met because she had general anesthesia.

3. Statement by Mrs. G., "I was a failure in delivery."

Plan

The nursing plan is to promote a positive self-concept through a positive acceptance of the childbirth experience.

Intervention

Nursing Interventions	Rationale	Outcome Criteria
1. Encourage the patient to discuss her labor and delivery experience	Discussion of the birth experience allows the mother to absorb and consolidate her experience into a positive part of herself. This is a normal part of the taking-in phase and should be promoted (Rubin, 1961).	Patient will be able to evaluate her labor and delivery experience, and the nurse has a better understanding of what this experience means to the patient.
2. Encourage the patient to discuss unmet expectations of labor and delivery.	Ventilation of unmet needs helps the patient progress through the taking-in phase and regain a positive sense of self (Rubin, 1961).	Patient will acknowledge the use of general anesthesia as a necessary alternative method.

Nursing Interventions (Cont'd)	Rationale (Cont'd)	Outcome Criteria (Cont'd)
3. Help Mrs. G. identify goals of safety for herself and the baby at delivery.	Mrs. G. will be able to accept circumstances of her delivery after considering the need for safe delivery of the baby.	Will accept measures used to provide a safe delivery and healthy baby.

Evaluation

After discussing her birth experience, Mrs. G. seemed able to accept the need for general anesthesia. She seemed to be progressing well through the taking-in phase.

––––––––––––––––– NURSING DIAGNOSIS –––––––––––––––––

Alterations in uterine involution associated with decreased uterine tone.

Assessment

Significant data for this second nursing diagnosis included:

1. Boggy uterus.
2. Uterus at level of umbilicus.
3. Moderate amount of lochia rubra.
4. B.P. 120/70, P. 64.
5. Gravida 1, Para 1.
6. First postpartal day.

Plan

The nursing plan in this situation is to improve uterine tone to facilitate uterine involution.

Intervention

Nursing Interventions	Rationale	Outcome Criteria
1. Massage the fundus until firm to stimulate uterine muscle contractions and increase uterine tone. Teach patient uterine massage.	Uterine massage will increase uterine tone and decrease lochia flow (Reid, 1972).	The uterus will become contracted and firm; patient does uterine massage to increase uterine tone.

Nursing Interventions (Cont'd)	*Rationale (Cont'd)*	*Outcome Criteria (Cont'd)*
2. Encourage frequent voidings to prevent bladder from interfering with involution.	After delivery, the sensation to void is frequently diminished.	Bladder will not be distended. First three voidings equal 500 cc.

Evaluation

Mrs. G. demonstrates the proper method of uterine massage. After massage, the uterus becomes firm. Fundus decreases at the rate of one finger breadth each day. Lochia flow decreases as uterus becomes firmer.

————————————— **NURSING DIAGNOSIS** —————————————

Fear of breast-feeding related to a lack of knowledge and experience with the breast-feeding process.

Assessment

Significant data for this nursing diagnosis included:

1. Mrs. G.'s lack of understanding of the process of milk production; she says her breasts are too small.

2. Mrs. G.'s many questions about the mechanics of breast-feeding.

3. Mrs. G.'s distraught facial expression, nervous hand movements, and statements such as "I don't think I can do this."

Plan

The nurse plans to alleviate Mrs. G.'s fear by increasing her knowledge of and positive experiences with breast-feeding.

Intervention

Nursing Interventions	*Rationale*	*Outcome Criteria*
1. Instruct the patient about the anatomy of the breast and the formation of breast milk.	Understanding the concepts of breast milk formation will promote an understanding of the lactation process and facilitate successful breast-feeding (Zeigel and Cranley, 1979).	Patient understands basic anatomy of the breast and is able to discuss breast milk formation.

Nursing Interventions (Cont'd)	Rationale (Cont'd)	Outcome Criteria (Cont'd)
2. Discuss positioning of the mother and baby for breast-feeding.	If the mother assumes a position that is comfortable for her and a position in which the baby is able to suckle, this promotes the letdown reflex. Proper positioning is important in avoiding the frustration of not being able to get the baby to the breast (Zeigel and Cranley, 1979).	Mother will be able to assume a comfortable position for breast-feeding.
3. Teach Mrs. G. methods of getting baby to and from the breast.	If the mother uses proper technique in putting the baby to and from the breast, this helps avoid sore nipples caused by excessive negative pressure (Iffrig, 1968).	Mother gains confidence in her ability to position baby for feeding and removes the baby from the breast without nipple damage.
4. Teach the mother alternate massage to ensure complete emptying of the breasts.	Alternate massage allows for complete emptying of the breast by facilitating the flow of milk from the alveoli to the milk reservoirs. This helps prevent engorgement (Iffrig, 1968).	The entire breast will be softened after the feeding, indicating complete emptying.
5. Teach mother techniques to increase her supply of breast milk. Instruct mother that complete emptying of the breast is the stimulus that causes increased milk production. If the breast is not emptied, less milk is produced.	For successful breast-feeding, the mother will need to know methods of adjusting her milk supply (Iffrig, 1968).	Patient verbalizes understanding of techniques to increase or decrease milk production.
6. Teach mother proper care of breasts.	If proper care of breast is observed, this will help prevent sore nipples and complications with breast-feeding (Iffrig, 1968).	Patient verbalizes and demonstrates proper care of the breasts.

Evaluation

The baby is receiving 90 to 100 grams of milk at each feeding as demonstrated by weights before and after feeding. He is sleeping two and a half to three hours after each feeding. Mrs. G. feels comfortable about her ability to breast feed. Her breasts are soft and empty; her nipples are not cracked.

_____ NURSING DIAGNOSIS _____

Altered self-definition in social roles associated with changed life style following birth of baby.

Assessment

Significant data for this nursing diagnosis included:

1. Mrs. G. states that having a baby will change her life style.
2. Having a baby will cause alterations in roles and may cause some role conflict (Clark, 1978).
3. Mrs. G. states she will miss her friends and the students at school.
4. Mrs. G.'s husband is discouraging her return to work.

Plan

The nurse will encourage in Mrs. G. the development of a new self-definition incorporating the altered life style changes.

Intervention

Nursing Interventions	Rationale	Outcome Criteria
1. Encourage discussion that relates to Mrs. G.'s feelings of loss.	Loss of independence is usually part of early motherhood. Mrs. G. is experiencing the loss of her previous role as a teacher and the support and gratification that was associated with her work. This loss can be partially compensated for if there is sufficient feedback to the mother in her new role (Clark and Affonso, 1979).	Mrs. G. feels comfortable in discussing feelings about role losses.
2. Allow husband and wife time to ventilate feelings regarding changes in life style.	Discussion of changes in life style allows the couple to make anticipatory plans for adapting to their new life with their baby (Duvall, 1971).	Parents discuss adaptations that they will be making in the immediate future to accommodate their new baby.

Nursing Interventions (Cont'd)	Rationale (Cont'd)	Outcome Criteria (Cont'd)
3. Give praise for accomplishments in mothering tasks.	Praise for accomplishments facilitates the taking on of the new role (Rubin, 1975).	Mother feels confident in her ability to give infant care.
4. Promote development of parent-infant attachment through frequent physical contact of mother and baby.	Positive attachment to the newborn is important for his survival because he is dependent upon the parents to meet all of his needs.	Parental care of the infant reflects a positive parent-infant bond.

Evaluation

Mrs. G. begins to work through her feelings related to the change in life style and role. Each day the mother increases tactile communication and eye to eye contact with her infant. Mrs. G. states she feels better about not returning to work; staying home will give her more time with the baby and allow her to breast-feed for a longer period of time.

——————————————— NURSING DIAGNOSIS ———————————————

Lack of knowledge and skill in baby care associated with child care inexperience.

Assessment

Significant data for this nursing diagnosis included:

1. This is Mr. and Mrs. G.'s first baby.
2. Mr. and Mrs. G. ask many questions regarding baby care.

Plan

The nursing plan is to increase the parents' knowledge and skills of baby care.

Intervention

Nursing Interventions	Rationale	Outcome Criteria
1. Examine baby and review findings with parents.	Discussion of the baby's physical examination encourages the parents to ask questions and learn about the characteristics of their newborn. This also facilitates the claiming process (Clausen and co-workers, 1976).	Parents observe the newborn's examination and feel free to ask questions about their baby.
2. Discuss signs and symptoms of common illnesses in the newborn: elevated temperature, diarrhea, continuous crying, irritability, skin rashes, abnormal breathing.	If the parents become aware of symptoms of illness in their baby, they will know when to call the physician.	Parents discuss symptoms that would indicate the need to consult with a physician.
3. Teach parents how to give the baby a bath and allow time for them to try it.	New parents often feel uncomfortable in giving their baby a bath for the first time. The nurse is able to assist the parents in feeling comfortable in caring for their infant. This reinforces the mother's feeling that she is able to care for her baby (Pillitteri, 1977).	Parents feel comfortable in giving care to their new baby.
4. Discuss the need for infant stimulation and encourage the parents to talk and play with their baby.	Playing and talking to the baby stimulates the baby's physical, emotional, and language development (Klaus and Kennell, 1976).	Parents understand the need for infant stimulation to promote development.
5. Discuss infant nutrition, emphasizing the correlation between the quality of maternal breast milk and maternal nutrition. Encourage the delay of introduction of solids to the infant until the parents discuss this with their pediatrician.	Maternal nutrition affects the quality of the breast milk. Early introduction of solids may stimulate allergy development and obesity (Thomas and co-workers, 1970).	The mother understands the need for proper nutrition to produce high quality milk. She also understands the relationship between early introduction of solids and the development of food allergy and obesity.

Nursing Interventions (Cont'd)	Rationale (Cont'd)	Outcome Criteria (Cont'd)
6. Encourage a four week examination for the infant and a six week postpartum checkup for the mother.	Assessment of the health of the mother and baby assures the detection of any complications (Clausen and coworkers, 1976).	Mother has an appointment for the baby's examination and her six week postpartal checkup.

Evaluation

During this taking-hold phase the mother was very receptive to health teaching. She demonstrated confidence in handling and feeding the baby. The mother assumes the enface position (looking into the baby's eyes) when holding the baby. The father is doing a significant amount of touching, holding, and care-giving. The parents relate to the baby by his name at all times and give him much tactile stimulation.

Summary of Mrs. G.'s Progress

By the morning of discharge, the patient has had an opportunity to receive baby care and breast-feeding instructions. Postpartal examination revealed the process of involution to be within normal limits, as were breasts, perineum, and vaginal discharge. Mrs. G. was breast-feeding her infant without difficulty. Manual expression and alternate massage were demonstrated by the patient. Patient understands proper diet for a lactating mother. The G.'s have anticipated adjustments that they will make in relation to the arrival of their new infant. The nurse gave Mrs. G. her phone number and encouraged her to call if she had difficulties. The nurse plans to phone Mrs. G. three days after discharge to assess her adjustment to her new life style and role.

References

Anderson, R., and Carter, I.: *Human Behavior in the Social Environment.* Chicago, Aldine Publishing Company, 1974.

Barnes, A.: *Intra-uterine Development.* Philadelphia, Lea and Febiger, 1968.

Caplan, G.: *Concepts of Mental Health and Consultation Application: Public Health Social Work,* Washington, D.C., U.S. Department of Health, Education, and Welfare, 1970.

Clark, A.: *Culture, Childbearing, Health Professionals.* Philadelphia, F.A. Davis Company, 1978.

Clark, A., and Affonso, D.: *Childbearing: A Nursing Perspective,* 2nd ed. Philadelphia, F.A. Davis Company, 1979.

Clausen, J., Flock, M., and Ford, B.: *Maternity Nursing Today,* 2nd ed. New York, McGraw-Hill Book Co., 1976.

Danforth, D., ed.: *Textbook of Obstetrics and Gynecology,* 3rd ed. New York, Harper & Row, 1977.

Duvall, E.: *Family Development.* Philadelphia, J.B. Lippincott Co., 1971.

Erikson, E.H.: *Childhood and Society*, 2nd ed. New York, W.W. Norton & Co., 1963.

Fawcett, J.: Body image and the pregnant couple. *American Journal of Maternal Child Nursing*, 3:227, 1978.

Friedman, E.: *Labor: Clinical Evaluation and Management*, 2nd ed. New York, Appleton-Century-Crofts, 1978.

Goodlin, R.: Importance of the lateral position during labor. *Obstetrics and Gynecology*, 37:698, 1971.

Hon, E.: *An Introduction to Fetal Heart Rate Monitoring*, 2nd ed. New Haven, Harty Press, 1975.

Iffrig, Sr., M.C.: Body image in pregnancy: Its relation to nursing functions. *Nursing Clinics of North America*, 7:631, 1972.

Iffrig, Sr., M.C.: Nursing care and success in breast feeding. *Nursing Clinics of North America*, 3:345, 1968.

Jensen, M., Benson, R., and Bobak, I.: *Maternity Care: The Nurse and the Family.* St. Louis, The C.V. Mosby Company, 1977.

Kennell, J.H., and Rolnick, A.R.: Discussing problems in newborn babies with their parents. *Pediatrics, 26:*832, 1960.

Kilker, R., and Wilkerson, B.: Assessment: 8-point postpartum assessment. *Nursing, 73*, 3:56, 1973.

Klaus, M., and Kennell, J.: *Maternal Infant Bonding.* St. Louis, The C.V. Mosby Company, 1976.

McConnell, O.L., and Daston, P.G.: Body image changes in pregnancy. *Journal of Projective Techniques, 25:*451, 1961.

Olds, S., London, M., Ladewig, P., and Davidson, S.: *Obstetric Nursing.* Reading, MA., Addison-Wesley Publishing Company, 1980.

Oxorn, H., and Foote, W.: *Human Labor and Birth*, 3rd ed. New York, Appleton-Century-Crofts, 1980.

Pillitteri, A.: *Nursing Care of the Growing Family.* Boston, Little, Brown and Company, 1977.

Pritchard, J., and MacDonald, P.: *Williams Obstetrics*, 15th ed. New York, Appleton-Century-Crofts, 1976.

Reeder, S., Mastroianne, L., Martin, W., and Fitzpatrick, E.: *Maternity Nursing*, 13th ed. Philadelphia, J.B. Lippincott Company, 1976.

Reid, D., Ryan, K., and Benirschke, K.: *Principles and Management of Human Reproduction.* Philadelphia, W.B. Saunders Co., 1972.

Rubin, R.: Puerperal change. *Nursing Outlook, 9:*753, 1961.

Rubin, R.: Cognitive style of pregnancy. *American Journal of Nursing, 70:*502, 1970.

Rubin, R.: Maternal tasks in pregnancy. *Maternal Child Nursing Journal, 75:*143, 1975.

Tanner, L.: Assessing the needs of new mothers in the postpartum unit. *In* Duffey, M.A.: *Current Concepts in Clinical Nursing*, vol. 3. St. Louis, The C.V. Mosby Company, 1971.

Thomas, A., Chess, S., and Birch, H.: The origin of personality. *Scientific American, 223:* 102, 1970.

Wiedenbach, E.: *Family Centered Maternity Nursing.* New York, G.P. Putnam's Sons, 1967.

Williams, S.R.: *Nutrition and Diet Therapy*, 2nd ed. St. Louis, The C.V. Mosby Company, 1973.

Woman-Infant-Child Supplemental Feeding Program. Washington, D.C., U.S. Department of Agriculture, Food and Nutritional Service, 1978.

Ziegel, E., and Cranley, M.: *Obstetric Nursing*, 7th ed. New York, Macmillan Company, Inc., 1979.

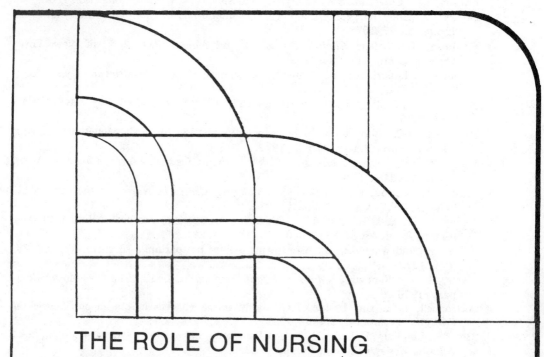

THE ROLE OF NURSING DIAGNOSIS IN THE CARE OF A HOSPITALIZED ADOLESCENT AND HIS FAMILY

12

Helen R. DiCroce, R.N., B.S.N., M.S.N.

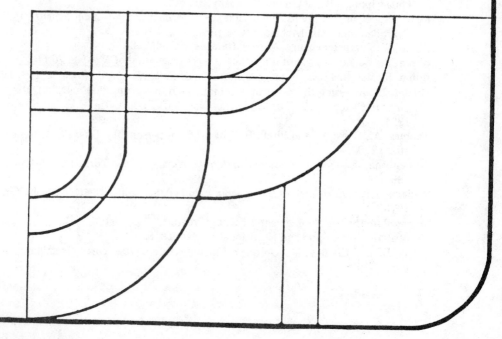

Through establishment of accurate nursing diagnoses, nurses make a significant difference to a sick child and his family during a period of hospitalization. By application of knowledge from a broad-based scientific background, the professional nurse is in a unique position to explore adaptive physiological, psychological, social, cultural, and developmental dimensions of hospitalized children and their parents and to identify significant responses which might require nursing intervention. The assessment process of identifying unique differences in a child and his family's responses to a given health situation yields data that, when analyzed and synthesized, lead to the nursing diagnoses. The nursing diagnoses are the bases for determining nursing plans, actions, and evaluations.

A universal goal of nurses caring for hospitalized children and their families is to provide quality care that insures them the least possible stress associated with the hospitalization experience. Operationalizing this goal for an individual child and his family is the focus of this chapter. The patient study presents a chronically ill adolescent boy admitted to the hospital for elective surgery, which he hopes will provide him with a sphere of independence previously unknown to him.

Hospitalization of an adolescent creates stress, not only for him, but for the family as well. Established living patterns of a family are changed when the need for hospitalization disrupts the security of familiar routines. Family dynamics are altered when trusted and familiar persons are not available. When increased time allotment and emotional investment of the mother are required by one child because of his separation from home, all family members are affected. Mothers create the emotional climate between themselves and their children (Spitz, 1966). Thus, *she is the single most influential factor in the stability of the family*.

Duvall (1971) attests to the universality of the difficulties families experience, even under the most favorable circumstances, in adequately meeting the growth needs of all members of different ages, sexes, interests, and personalities. Change in established living patterns forces a reorganization of the family as a social system. Roles have to be reassigned, status positions shifted, values reoriented, and needs met through new channels (LeMasters, 1965). The family can survive only if all its members, adults and children, receive support, acceptance, and the opportunity for working through the developmental tasks that each must achieve in order to move into the next stage of their development (Duvall, 1971).

The professional nurse, cognizant of these family needs, directs her energies not only to the hospitalized adolescent, but to the family as well. Through a family-centered approach, the nurse is able to assess the extent and limitations of the family's adaptive capacities and resources; such assessment data form the bases for nursing diagnoses. The plan of care includes mobilizing all available resources by utilizing the composite strengths of all family members, for it is this *composite* strength that constitutes a given family's resources in adapting to stress (Riddle, 1973). Nursing interventions include specific measures to mobilize resources, including providing a place for the mother to rest in the hospital or modifying hospital routines and policies to accommodate visiting by various family members. Evaluation, the last step of the nursing process, is likewise directed toward the family as well as the client because of their important role in the client's progress.

The educational preparation of the professional nurse includes the following areas of knowledge that are needed for family-centered nursing: developmental theories of families and individuals, leadership, management, communication, and group dynamics. In practice, this knowledge is operationalized only through purposeful, systematic application of it by the professional nurse to the health care needs of individual patients and families. This knowledge, coupled with the understanding of basic sciences and medical therapies for specific health needs, is an essential prerequisite needed to arrive at accurate nursing diagnoses. Without the use of all this knowledge, the assessment of patient and family needs is incomplete, and accurate nursing diagnoses are impossible.

CLIENT SITUATION: RANDY, A CHRONICALLY ILL ADOLESCENT

Randy A., 16 years old, was admitted to the medical center's pediatric hospital on December 17 for elective surgical implant of a prosthetic urinary sphincter on December 19. He was born with a myelomeningocele and accompanying hydrocephalus. Both were treated surgically shortly after birth.

Myelomeningocele is a nervous system anomaly characterized by incomplete fusion of one or more vertebral arches with impaired development of the spinal cord. There is subsequent cystic distention of the meninges with the presence of nerve tissue within the sac. Surgical treatment of myelomeningocele is closure of the sac, a procedure which does not correct the neural defect but only removes the protrusion. The individual has permanent neurological deficit to body parts affected by the damaged spinal cord. Hydrocephalus (increased cerebrospinal fluid pressure) occurs in 75 per cent of these cases. This is controlled surgically through shunting of excess fluid (Steele, 1977).

Neurogenic bladder is one result of myelomeningocele and one factor in the chain of events which leads to kidney damage, the major life-threatening complication of myelomeningocele. From birth, special procedures are used to facilitate adequate bladder emptying, such as Credé technique, intermittent catheterization, and surgical urinary diversion. A more recent treatment of urinary incontinence involves the implantation of a prosthetic urinary sphincter. This therapy has the advantage of providing the individual, male or female, with volitional urinary control. The Scott sphincter (Fig. 12–1) consists of a reservoir, an inflatable cuff, and a pump. The reservoir contains radiopaque fluid that is pumped into the cuff and then back again. The cuff encircles the urethra and when inflated produces concentric pressure, like a sphincter, against the urethra (Scott and coworkers, 1973). In males the pump is implanted in the scrotum and in females in the labia majora. When the patient wants to empty his bladder he releases the fluid from the cuff into the reservoir, which has been implanted in the abdominal cavity. After bladder emptying, he inflates the cuff again, producing the effects of a functioning sphincter.

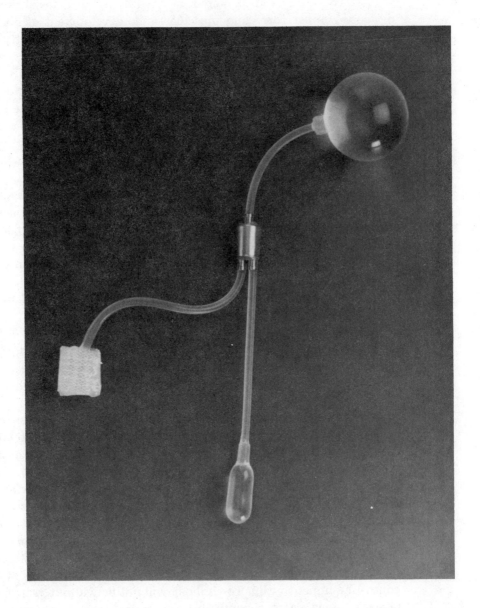

Figure 12–1 Scott sphincter.

Assessment

Randy's birth defect presented him with major life challenges which he has met with varying degrees of success. He has minimal use of his lower extremities and a neurogenic bladder. Frequent hospitalizations for surgical and medical treatments have been a part of his life. Bladder and bowel regimes, physical therapy, brace and crutch walking, psychological adjustment to his physically deformed body, and successful social and academic adaptation at school are facets of his ongoing efforts in adjusting to his defects.

At 16 he is a dark-haired boy with pleasing facial features, well-developed upper torso and muscular underdevelopment of his body below the waist. Randy is in generally good health though slightly overweight. Pubescent changes have given a deep masculine quality to his voice and there is evidence of beginning facial hair. He walks with the aid of braces and crutches. His denim clothing is typical of casual rural living, and their quality reflects moderately affluent economic resources. Socially, he demonstrates familiarity with the hospital unit personnel, although his response to individuals ranges noticeably from pleasantness to hostility. He expresses preference for some of the nurses; this is evidenced by his calling them by name.

The interview between Randy and the primary care nurse reveals that he had an active role in electing to have a Scott sphincter implanted. He has high hopes for the resulting bladder control and consequent independence that the procedure will afford him. Randy's career plans are not firmly established, but he verbalizes the importance of education in preparing for employment and economic independence. He attends the local public high school where he is a junior. Academically, he is a "B" student who favors mathematics.

Randy lives with his parents, his brother, John, and his sister, Melissa. They live on a large ranch 95 miles from the medical center. His father breeds and trains race horses, and Randy speaks knowledgeably about the subject. His admiration for his father is apparent, as well as his closeness to his mother, brother, and sister. His greatest desire is to have his own horse to train. He spontaneously offers the reason why this is impossible explaining that the horse could mistake his crutch for a training stick, thereby making him vulnerable to attack by the horse. He states with a tone of defeat in his voice that this potential danger would worry his mother and that this is not a realistic goal. Another indication of Randy's self-concept surfaced when he asked the nurse to replace a cover that had slipped from the lower part of his legs saying, "Who wants to look at them, they are so ugly."

Randy's surgery was purposely scheduled for the Christmas holidays in order to take advantage of the school break. Being away from home and friends for Christmas is compensated for by the anticipation of the bladder control he hopes to gain. The holiday will not be without visits from friends, however, since several schoolmates plan to visit Randy after he has recovered from the surgery.

Randy's mother accompanied him to the medical center. From past experience with Mrs. A., the nurse knows that she is a 41 year old woman in good health, who has an active role in operating the ranch with her husband. The husband is 42 and healthy. Mrs. A. stated that Randy requested to have his surgery performed during the holiday period. His wish was considered without hesitation, since both she and her husband knew that during the following spring Randy would be faced with several social functions, and they wanted him to have the advantage of the increased freedom that would be provided by the artificial sphincter. She verbalized concern for Randy regarding sexual maturity and all of its emotional awakenings.

She appeared well informed and confident in her ability to meet the challenges of this hospitalization with the same composure with which she had handled all the previous treatments, setbacks, and surgeries of the past sixteen years. She indicated that they had no financial worries at this time and that family members were supportive of each other.

As in the past, Mr. A. would be present on the day of surgery and on the first post-operative day only. After this, it would be necessary for him to return to his responsibilities at the ranch. Mrs. A. arranged to be free to visit Randy more frequently throughout his hospitalization.

Mrs. A.'s conversation turned to her other two children. Melissa, her 3½ year old daughter, seemed confused by the fact that Randy had to go away to a hospital when he wasn't sick. She remembered when he was hospitalized recently for treatment of cellulitis and could easily relate to the idea of having his "sore fixed."

John, 14 years old, grew up with Randy and seems to accept Randy's handicap as a fact of life. His needs have not been neglected, and Mrs. A. speaks admiringly of John's generosity towards Randy in terms of time and patience. This brotherly assistance occurs sometimes at the expense of companionship with his own friends, who are not always as understanding. She and her husband provide John with opportunities to be free from the felt responsiblity towards Randy. They feel these opportunities are insurance against later resentment that could otherwise develop. John recently verbalized to his father his feelings of sadness and hopelessness for Randy as he himself experiences early heterosexual interests. He knows how much acceptance is dependent on physical attractiveness during adolescence and how Randy might be affected by this and feel rejected.

By the completion of her conversations with Randy and his mother, the nurse had a greater understanding of the complexities involved in the A.'s family unit, which overtly appeared well equipped to handle this hospitalization based on its past experiences and the member's close support of each other. This knowledge led the nurse to understand that her nursing care for Randy and her relationships with his parents encompassed much more than pre- and post-operative activities and teaching the mechanics of the Scott sphincter. Ongoing assessment of the entire family's needs would be the only basis for day to day and hour to hour nursing decisions. The nurse thought of Randy's request to be cared for by certain nurses and recalled his hostile reaction to some of the unit personnel and his friendliness towards others.

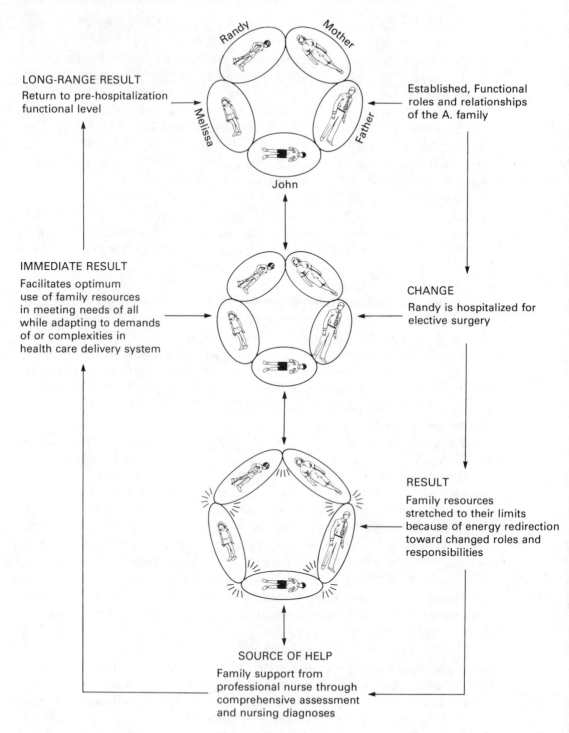

LONG-RANGE RESULT
Return to pre-hospitalization functional level

Established, Functional roles and relationships of the A. family

IMMEDIATE RESULT
Facilitates optimum use of family resources in meeting needs of all while adapting to demands of or complexities in health care delivery system

CHANGE
Randy is hospitalized for elective surgery

RESULT
Family resources stretched to their limits because of energy redirection toward changed roles and responsibilities

SOURCE OF HELP
Family support from professional nurse through comprehensive assessment and nursing diagnoses

She thought of how all of the collected information could be utilized to provide effective care for Randy and his family and how co-workers might be alerted to the effect that each had on Randy. She also considered the unit rules and regulations and whether or not they were realistic in meeting the needs of hospitalized adolescents.

A remark made to Randy by another nurse provided additional information about his attitude toward the staff. In a playful and teasing manner the other nurse said, "Well, I see you couldn't stay away. Since you like it here so much, I hope you won't be so grouchy this time." Randy appeared visibly upset by the remark and turned to go to his room without responding.

During previous hospitalizations, Randy had been cared for by many nurses. Their brief and fragmented experiences with him did not allow them to know him or his mother well enough to gain an understanding of their responses and whether or not those responses were appropriate. What was perceived as "grouchiness" by the one nurse was actually Randy's need to be alone to deal with a new level of insight he had gained about himself and what his handicap meant to long-range life plans. His response to the nurse's teasing indicated that whatever produced his behavior at the time was not viewed as unimportant to him. From this, the nurse concluded that a small nucleus of nurses who would care for him during the time of his hospitalization would provide Randy with the opportunity to develop confidence and trust in them. They could then be resources for him to share more of his concerns, knowing that those concerns would be given the respect and importance they deserved.

Randy's physical examination revealed:

1. Normocephalic: hydrocephalus successfully treated after birth.

2. Full function and strength of upper extremities.

3. Lungs clear, heart regular.

4. Back reveals a healed area over the lumbar spine where the defect has been grafted and closed.

5. Lower extremities:
   a. Skin well cared for and intact, but no sensation present below knees.
   b. Active flexion and adduction of hips; essentially no abduction or extension of hips.
   c. Weak active extension of knees.
   d. Lower extremities flaccid, given exceptions noted above.

Laboratory tests are normal with the exception of data indicating a chronic urinary tract infection.

Nursing Diagnoses

Five nursing diagnoses were formulated based on the assessment data obtained pre-operatively by the nurse in conjunction with the knowledge she possessed about Randy as an individual, adolescent, and family member, the expected pre- and post- operative outcome of his surgery, and the impact of the health care delivery system on Randy.

Randy's nursing diagnoses include the following:

1. At risk for urinary leakage related to bladder distention following surgery.

2. At risk for post-operative infection related to poor circulation as a result of the myelomeningocele.

3. Negative self-image related to perceived physical unattractiveness.

4. Isolation related to hospital environment.

5. Altered family relationships related to hospitalization.

Each of these nursing diagnoses will be discussed individually as the nurse develops a plan of care, determines interventions to achieve the plan, and specifies criteria that will determine the degree to which the plan of care is successful.

_____ NURSING DIAGNOSIS _____

At risk for urinary leakage related to bladder distention following surgery.

Plan

Intervention

Plan	Interventions	Rationale	Outcome Criteria
Prevent bladder distention by teaching Randy about:			
1. Scott sphincter	Secure Scott sphincter from O.R. for Randy to see and handle. Fill the reservoir with water and demonstrate how the liquid is pumped into the cuff and then returned to the reservoir.	Teaching facilitates a change in behavior, a necessity for the successful operation of Randy's Scott sphincter. Since the entire mechanism is internal when implanted, it is best explained by visualizing its components and workings.	Randy will demonstrate the operation of the pumping mechanism of the Scott sphincter.
2. Post-operative expectations.	Provide Randy with information about what he can expect to feel and experience after surgery:	It is important for Randy to know what to anticipate after surgery, and much of it depends on the degree of	Randy will relate his experiences as normal or abnormal based on information given.

Plan (Cont'd)	Interventions (Cont'd)	Rationale (Cont'd)	Outcome Criteria (Cont'd)
	(a) a temporary burning of the urethra caused by the surgical procedure itself; (b) bladder spasms, varied in intensity, depending on his bladder capacity for contractility; (c) pain for a 3-week post-operative period when pumping the mechanism.	sensation he has. Such knowledge will allow him to discriminate between what is normal and abnormal.	
3. Complete bladder emptying	Review the proper procedure for the Credé technique. Explain the effects of various factors such as fluid intake, activity, and diet on bladder functioning.	Incomplete bladder emptying is one cause for incontinence between pumpings.	Randy will demonstrate understanding of the new role that the Credé technique plays by repeating the information that the nurse has given him. He will describe the various factors that affect bladder function.
4. Sources of increased intra-abdominal pressure.	Explain that intermittent leaking may result from change in position, coughing, laughing, sneezing, distended bowel, and straining.	Adequacy of the Scott sphincter is affected by increased intra-abdominal pressure.	Randy will list causes of leaking from intra-abdominal pressure.
	Take measures to maintain bowel regime, for example, use of stool softeners.	A distended bowel increases intra-abdominal pressure.	Regular bowel evacuation will occur.

Evaluation

At the time of Randy's discharge he was well on his way to controlling and managing the operation of the Scott sphincter. Episodes of urinary leakage were diminishing in frequency and volume, and his progress was within expectations. He was highly motivated to continue his efforts to establish complete freedom from leakage. He seemed very proud of his newly realized independence.

_____ NURSING DIAGNOSIS _____

At risk for post-operative infection related to poor circulation as a result of the myelomeningocele.

Plan

Intervention

Plan	Interventions	Rationale	Outcome Criteria
Prevent infection by decreasing number of personnel contacts.	Daily dressing changes will be done by the same nurse who evaluates the condition of the suture line. A record of the incisional area will be made after each dressing change with particular note of any changes since the previous evaluation. Condition of the suture line will be reported to the nurse responsible for Randy for the following shift.	As a result of Randy's neurological deficit in the operative area, he has markedly diminished sensation. Observation of the site is the primary method of monitoring the suture line condition. Changes can be recognized early if the same nurse performs this function daily.	Satisfactory healing will occur.

Plan (Cont'd)	Interventions (Cont'd)	Rationale (Cont'd)	Outcome Criteria (Cont'd)
Prevent infection by maintaining aseptic techniques at suture line.	Maintain strict sterile field during dressing change.	Diminished circulation makes the operative site more vulnerable to infection.	No evidence of infection of the suture line. Negative culture reports.
	Use topical medications ordered for the suture line accurately and on time.	With diminished circulation, antibiotics for topical and systemic use are important adjuncts to prevent infection when the skin surface has been interrupted.	
	Administer systemic antibiotics accurately and on time.		
	Culture the suture line according to the established schedule using proper technique.	Identification of a pathological organism can be determined by culture.	
Increase circulation to operative site.	Use a 25 watt bulb and place the lamp 12 inches from the operative site.	Proper amount of external heat improves circulation.	Evidence of healing.
	Stay with Randy during the 20 minute treatment.	With diminished sensation there is increased danger of burns with use of heat lamp.	No evidence of tissue damage caused by use of heat lamp.

Evaluation

Randy's post-operative course progressed satisfactorily without occurrence of infection. Heat lamp treatments to increase circulation proved to be effective, and there was no indication of burns to surrounding tissue.

_____ **NURSING DIAGNOSIS** _____

Negative self image related to perceived physical unattractiveness.

Plan

Intervention

Plan	Interventions	Rationale	Outcome Criteria
Create a climate for expression of positive and negative feelings.	Allow time for establishment of a therapeutic relationship between Randy and the nurse.	Spontaneity on Randy's part is dependent on a relationship in which there is mutual respect and trust.	There will be increased spontaneity on Randy's part in confiding in a few well known and trusted nurses.
	Accept his expressions of hostility without value judgments.	It should be anticipated that Randy must first test his caretakers before being able to disclose important feelings. He will need to know that his feelings will be considered important and respected.	With establishment of trust, Randy's aggression will be directed in more constructive outlets.
	Accept Randy's expression of disgust for his body appearance.	Randy's feelings about himself must be acknowledged by him and others as honest and legitimate expressions of disappointment at the loss of physical wholeness.	Randy will continue to express feelings about himself.
	Acknowledge Randy's accomplishments by specifying his obvious assets and creating opportunities for him to define his accomplishments.	Recognition of past accomplishments reinforces self-esteem.	Randy will acknowledge his accomplishments.

Evaluation

As Randy became accustomed to "his" nurse he became more open with her. He confided how much he was hurt and frustrated by comments made to him by others who did not even try to understand his feelings about himself. As time went on he expanded his trusting association to selected others while remaining distant toward those he saw as a threat to him.

_____ **NURSING DIAGNOSIS** _____

Isolation related to the hospital environment.

Plan

Intervention

Plan	Interventions	Rationale	Outcome Criteria
Encourage visits by friends.	Make necessary arrangements for friends to spend several hours when they come to visit rather than asking them to leave when regular visiting hours are over. Provide a place where all visitors can spend time with Randy together rather than limiting visitation to two persons at a time. Suggest that phone calls be planned on days when visitors are not expected.	Peers are highly significant to adolescents. Modifications in established policies are desirable because of the travel time and distance involved for Randy's visitors.	Randy will maintain contact with close friends. Randy and his friends will feel comfortable about special considerations afforded them.

Plan (Cont'd)	Interventions (Cont'd)	Rationale (Cont'd)	Outcome Criteria (Cont'd)
Encourage family's presence at times when Randy may most need their support.	Make arrangements for overnight stays for Mrs. A. including use of a shower and the hospital cafeteria for meals.	Basic necessities must be available when away from home.	Randy will not be left to handle new experiences alone.
	Arrange a Christmas holiday celebration with family.	Holiday seasons are, by tradition, occasions when families are together.	Randy and his family will experience a sense of joy and unity in being together.

Evaluation

Randy's happiest moments in the hospital seemed to occur during the visits of his many friends. He became much more cheerful while they were present, and it was clear that they were highly significant to him. They acted as a group and seemed totally sufficient unto themselves. These observations gave the nurse insight into Randy's social self away from the hospital situation. Such insight increased the nurse's confidence in him and made it possible to reinforce his actual accomplishments. Because of Randy's own strengths, the nurse was able to help him even further.

Mrs. A. was available to Randy before and after the surgical procedure, when the sphincter was first put into operation, and when he performed the operation of the sphincter for the first time himself. He did not elect to have her present in his room for some of these situations, but was undoubtedly supported by her availability.

Mrs. A. expressed satisfaction and appreciation for accommodations made in her behalf which made her overnight stay as comfortable as possible.

The family celebrated Christmas with Randy, exchanging gifts and enjoying a holiday dinner. Their sense of solidarity was evident, and they felt strong as a family unit.

_____ **NURSING DIAGNOSIS** _____

Altered family relationships caused by hospitalization.

Plan

Intervention

Plan	Interventions	Rationale	Outcome Criteria
Promote the maintenance of age-appropriate functioning of all family members.	Suggest that Mrs. A. spend time at home with Melissa.	Young pre-schoolers need opportunities to have the undivided attention of significant persons. Adequate time given to Melissa can prevent her making demands for time when Mrs. A. is needed at the hospital.	Mrs. A. and Randy will accept Melissa's legitimate need for attention from significant others.
	Suggest that John be provided with opportunities for social activities with peers.	Peer relationships are essential to John's development as they are to Randy's. Activities with peers should ease the disruption caused by Randy and Mrs. A. being away for so long.	John will behave in his normal fashion throughout Randy's hospitalization.
	Encourage Mr. and Mrs. A. to take time for leisure activity while Randy is hospitalized.	When family disruptions require assumption of others' workloads, a conscious effort is required to schedule leisure activities.	Randy's parents will engage in some leisure-time activity.

Evaluation

At the time of discharge there was no apparent breakdown in family relationships as a result of the hospitalization. Mrs. A. anticipated that time would be needed to reestablish pre-hospitalization roles.

SUMMARY

Nursing diagnoses are determined by analysis and synthesis of assessment data. Through the establishment of nursing diagnoses, specific goals are established for each unique situation. Day to day interpretation of all aspects of behavior and responses to care and validation of those interpretations serve as the bases for determining appropriate nursing interventions through which goals of care are accomplished. No formula exists that can be applied to others or even to the same patient over a period of time, since individuals' and families' capacities for adapting are ever changing.

By their very role, professional nurses are in a unique position to influence the kind and extent of care a patient will receive while hospitalized. In Randy's case, professional nurses were instrumental in providing optimal care through their organized and knowledgeable progression through the five-step nursing process.

The nursing diagnoses made on the bases of Randy's assessment data became the foundation for a plan of care that addressed the health care needs of Randy and his family. Nursing interventions were designed to achieve the ultimate goal of increased independence for Randy. Evaluation of those interventions indicated that the goal was indeed accomplished. Resolution of each of Randy's nursing diagnoses had occurred, and he returned to the community with a heightened degree and spirit of independence.

Acknowledgement is made to Michaela Hoy, Nurse Clinician, Department of Urology, Saint Louis University Medical School, for her contributions to nursing interventions in the care of patients with prosthetic urinary bladder sphincter implants.

References

Duvall, E.M.: *Family Development*. Philadelphia, J.B. Lippincott Co., 1971.

LeMasters, E.E.: Parenthood as Crisis. *In* H.J. Parad (ed.): *Crisis Intervention: Selected Readings*. New York, Family Service Association of America, 1965.

Riddle, I.: Caring for children and their families. *In* Anderson, E.H., Bergersen, B.S., Duffey, M., and Rose, M.H. (eds.): *Current Concepts in Clinical Nursing* (Vol. 4). St. Louis, The C.V. Mosby Company, 1973.

Scott, F.B., et al.: Treatment of urinary incontinence by implantable prosthetic sphincter. *Urology, 1:*252, 1973.

Spitz, R.A., and Cobliner, W.: *The First Year of Life*. New York, International Universities Press, Inc., 1966.

Steele, S.: *Nursing Care of the Child with Long Term Illness*, 2nd ed. New York, Appleton-Century-Crofts, 1977.

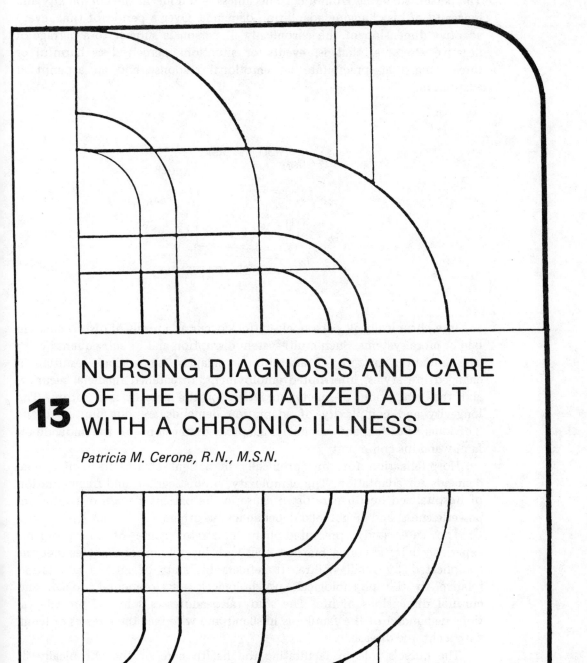

13

NURSING DIAGNOSIS AND CARE OF THE HOSPITALIZED ADULT WITH A CHRONIC ILLNESS

Patricia M. Cerone, R.N., M.S.N.

The person suffering from a chronic illness is unique in the complexity and longevity of his changing adaptation demands. Over a period of time, every adaptive dimension of the chronically ill person is subject to a barrage of negative stressors, that is, events or situations perceived as harmful or threatening that precipitate an emotional response and an attempt at adaptation.

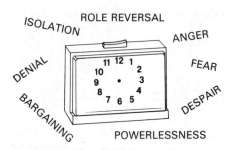

In a chronically ill person, alterations occur as a result of disturbances in one or more systems. Such multi-system disruption and its subsequent health care initiate a pattern of alteration in adaptive dimensions resulting in changed life styles, interrupted employment, threatened financial security, and the generation of many anxieties for the present and future. The longevity and complexity of adaptation demands are not limited to the individual, but expand to many adaptive dimensions of the individual's family and his community.

Hospitalization for the chronically ill patient creates its own special demands for adaptation. The complexity, sophistication, and fragmentation of hospitalized health care often cause in the patient a sense of confusion, powerlessness, and heightened dependency on others.

The case study presented here illustrates some of the problems experienced by a young married man with juvenile onset diabetes mellitus complicated by renal failure. It reflects his state of altered adaptation relative to the physiological, psychological, developmental, social, and cultural dimensions of life. The study also addresses some of the adaptations demanded of the family as husband and wife face the stresses of living with a chronic disease.

The nurse's role in facilitating the health care of the chronically ill hospitalized adult begins with the assessment of the patient's status within each of the five dimensions of adaptation. Past and present levels of functioning as well as access to internal and external resources constitute the data base from which nursing diagnoses can be formulated. Once nursing diagnoses are determined, direction is established for the remaining steps of the nursing process, that is, planning, intervention, and evaluation.

CLIENT SITUATION: Mr. T.J.

Mr. T.J., 31 years old, was hospitalized because of increasing renal dysfunction secondary to diabetes mellitus. He is scheduled for the creation of an arteriovenous (A.V.) fistula to be used for hemodialysis while he awaits a cadaver kidney for transplantation. Mr. J. was initially diagnosed as diabetic at age 13 and has a positive family history of diabetes mellitus for four generations. His medical history prior to four years ago is essentially non-significant to this hospitalization except for occasional episodes of hypoglycemia, syncope, and diabetic ketoacidosis associated with physical and psychological stress. Mr. J. has experienced visual deficits in both eyes as a result of diabetic retinopathy over the past three and a half years. These have been treated four times on an out-patient basis by photocoagulation. He now wears corrective lenses that allow him to operate an automobile and continue employment.

For the past two years he has been taking 500 mg. of methyldopa twice a day and 500 mg. of chlorothiazide daily for control of hypertension. Insulin-dependent since diagnosis, he has been regulated for most of his adult life by a combination of 60 U NPH Insulin at 7 a.m. and regular insulin on a sliding scale. Within the past sixteen months, insulin dosage changes and diet manipulations were necessary to treat increasing epidsodes of hypoglycemia. Satisfactory abatement of the hypoglycemic attacks was finally obtained with an American Diabetic Association (ADA) diet and an insulin schedule of regular insulin 10 U and NPH Insulin 20 U at 7 a.m. Other dietary restrictions of protein, fat, sodium, potassium, and fluid were recently initiated because of Mr. J.'s increasing renal dysfunction.

The admission interview by the nurse revealed some of the following information: Mr. J. states that he feels more tired than usual, especially toward the end of the day, yet sleep does not come easily. He finds it difficult to concentrate and repeatedly asks the same questions of the nurse. He believes his diabetes is improving, since he needs less insulin and no longer "spills" sugar.

Other pertinent history obtained by the nurse includes Mr. J.'s report of a metallic taste in his mouth and constant thirst, a productive cough in the morning, a loss of appetite, and inability to eat much at meal time. He acknowledges his rings, watch, and shoes feel tight, and he states he's gained ten pounds since his last doctor's appointment, three weeks ago. He complains of itching and a burning sensation along his back and legs. He reports calf pain, especially on the left, when he walks two blocks; he states that he usually has cold feet. He denies any history of foot infection.

Mr. J. admits to feeling angry about being in the hospital and being ill, yet he denies that his kidney disease will have any long-term effects on his life.

Mr. J. has been married for six years and lives with his wife in a suburban home. They have no children. Employed as a university instructor prior to his acute medical illness, he has been able to maintain his academic duties on a part-time basis until recently. He is active in church programs and professes a strong religious conviction since childhood. Mr. J.'s wife worked full time as a secretary in a small business, but recently lost her job because the company relocated.

Mr. J. is of German-English descent but admits no close cultural ties. His food preferences are German, and he enjoys the rousing music of the German culture. He acknowledges that his background is evident through his "stiff upper lip" approach to life.

Mr. J. reports some feelings of dissatisfaction with the level of achievement as an adult. Although he had secured a job, chosen a spouse, and settled into a home, he admitted that his illness "sometimes poses barriers to my reaching larger goals."

Admission examination of Mr. J. revealed a 170 pound male whose skin was a sallow color, dry, and scaling, but intact. His mouth contained several gingival lesions. His blood pressure was 174/119 mm Hg; pulse was 98/minute and regular; respirations were regular at 28/minute. Fine rales were heard at the base of both lungs.

Mr. J. had 3+ bilateral pitting edema in his lower extremities. Both legs were cool and pale with patches of brownish discoloration and trophic changes. Diminished vibratory sensation was present. Pedal pulses were decreased especially on the left; there was slow return of color to the nail beds.

Results of diagnostic studies indicated that Mr. J.'s electrocardiogram demonstrated peaked T waves associated with hyperkalemia. The chest film revealed bi-basilar infiltrates. Electromyography showed evidence of peripheral nerve damage. The blood and urine reports on Mr. J. (Tables 13–1 and 13–2), along with his medical history, demonstrated the clinical picture of renal failure as a complication of juvenile onset diabetes mellitus.

Three days following admission, Mr. J. underwent surgery for the creation of an A.V. fistula in his left forearm. He has at present been hospitalized twelve days and has received three hemodialysis treatments.

Since a future transplantation date is uncertain, the physician has discussed the feasibility of initiating home dialysis with Mrs. J. in attendance during treatments. Neither spouse has yet been able to discuss or come to a decision regarding this suggested treatment.

Mr. J. has not taken an active part in any of his treatments since admission. He has forced his wife into making whatever choices there were regarding his future, which she admits is unlike their previous pattern of relating. In reference to setting up hemodialysis at home, Mr. J. has stated that "it is not my decision to make, since the technical burden would be on my wife." The nursing staff has identified Mr. J.'s initial reaction to his current physical situation as regressive in nature with complete dependency on his wife. His wife acknowledges that his increased dependency is an initial method of coping with stress, but that with time, he regains self-sufficient behavior.

Mrs. J. confided to the nursing staff that she feels she "should learn to carry out the hemodialysis treatments at home, since it may mean the

Table 13–1 Laboratory Blood Work for Mr. J.

	Results	Normal Values
Chemistry		
Albumin	2.5 gm/100ml	3.2 –4.5 gm/100ml
Cholesterol	560 mg/100ml	150 – 250 mg/100ml
Chloride	101 mEq/L	95 – 103 mEq/L
CO_2 combining power	19 mEq/L	24 – 32 mEq/L
Creatinine	7.6 mg/100ml	0.6 –1.2 mg/100ml
Glucose (fasting)	160 mg/100ml	70 –110 mg/100ml
Potassium	6.2 mEq/L	3.8 – 5.0 mEq/L
Sodium	142 mEq/L	138 – 142 mEq/L
Total Proteins	4 gm/100ml	6.0 –7.8 gm/100ml
Urea Nitrogen	110 mg/100ml	10 – 20 mg/100ml
Hematology		
Hematocrit	30%	45 – 54%
Hemoglobin	9 gm/100ml	13.5 – 18 gm/100ml
WBC	8,000 cells/cu mm	5,000 – 10,000 cells/cu mm
Arterial Blood Gases (partial)		
pCO_2	20 mm Hg	35 – 40 mm Hg
pH	7.4	7.38 – 7.44

Table 13–2 Urinalysis for Mr. J.

	Results	Normal Values
Acetone	negative	negative
Glucose	negative	negative
pH	4.6	4.6 – 8.0
Protein	4+	negative
Specific Gravity	1.010	1.001 – 1.035

Microscopic examination: 1 to 2 white blood cells; occasional casts; negative for fat droplets.

difference between life and death for her husband." She has frequently voiced anger about the situation at hand. On more than one occasion she has said to several of the staff, "Why is this happening to us? We are good people!" Mrs. J. feels that communication with her husband is generally good, except when the subject of his health surfaces. Mrs. J. feels that her husband cannot accept some of his health limitations or make decisions about health-related matters.

Assessment data from Mr. and Mrs. J. were summarized, categorized, and labeled as nursing diagnostic statements. For the purposes of Mr. J.'s immediate hospitalized care, seven nursing diagnoses are presented. Each of them is discussed individually, describing the assessment data from which the diagnosis emerged, the plan of care suggested by the diagnosis, the interventions used to accomplish the plan, and the outcome criteria, the measures by which the nursing care will be evaluated. These seven nursing diagnoses include:

1. Risk for uncompensated metabolic acidosis associated with inadequate renal function.

2. Fluid overload secondary to inadequate renal function.

3. Risk for injury to the integument associated with impaired renal function.

4. Impaired peripheral circulation associated with diabetes mellitus.

5. Risk for infection secondary to damaged vascular system.

6. Insufficient dietary intake associated with altered renal function.

7. Anxiety related to severe and chronic alterations in health status.

_____ NURSING DIAGNOSIS _____

Risk for uncompensated metabolic acidosis associated with inadequate renal function.

Assessment

Significant data that formed the basis for this diagnosis included:

1. A history of increased fatigue and decreased ability to think clearly

2. A respiratory rate of 28 to 32/minute

3. Laboratory data that revealed the following:
   a. BUN = 110 mg per 100 ml   (normal 10 to 20 mg per 100 ml)
   b. Creatinine = 7.6 mg per 100 ml   (normal 0.6 to 1.2 mg per 100 ml)
   c. Serum K^+ = 6.2 mEq/L   (normal 3.8 to 5.5 mEq/L)
   d. pCO_2 = 20 mm Hg   (normal 35 to 40 mm Hg)
   e. Serum pH = 7.4   (normal 7.38 to 7.44)
   f. CO_2 combining power = 19
      mEq/L   (normal 24 to 32 mEq/L)

Plan

Intervention

Plan	Intervention	Rationale	Outcome Criteria
To support the state of compensated metabolic acidosis.	Teach about low potassium (K^+) diet.	Mr. J. needs to understand that continued intake of food containing K^+ would slowly poison him, since his kidneys cannot adequately eliminate this substance.	Able to name foods high in K^+. Maintains low K^+ diet. Pre-hemodialysis serum K^+ decreases to 6 mEq/L or less. No physical signs of increased muscle fatigue. Normal ECG tracing.
	Administration of the following medications: Aluminum gel *1* oz., four times a day; Sodium bicarbonate, 30 mEq, two times a day.	Control of acidosis secondary to renal failure may be achieved through oral administration of aluminum gel, which decreases fixed acids by binding phosphate in the intestines and helps to neutralize intestinal acid. The use of the base sodium bicarbonate helps to alleviate acidosis by restoring lost base. When sodium (Na^+) restrictions are concurrently being implemented, the Na^+ of sodium bicarbonate must be calculated into the dietary intake (Burrell and Burrell,	Remains in state of compensated metabolic acidosis according to serum pH, CO_2 combining power, and pCO_2. Serum sodium (Na^+) remains within normal limits.

Plan (Cont'd)	Intervention (Cont'd)	Rationale (Cont'd)	Outcome Criteria (Cont'd)
		1977; Hudak and coworkers, 1977).	
	Conduct hemodialysis treatments every other day.	In states of progressive renal failure, when the acidotic state is refractory to medication therapies alone, dialysis becomes necessary to rid the body of toxic levels of metabolic and catabolic wastes.	Gradual correction of serum electrolyte and chemical abnormalities.

Evaluation

No indication of hyperkalemia or decompensation of the state of metabolic acidosis was noted in Mr. J. The nursing staff was able to meet with Mr. J. and his wife twice weekly, at which time diet restrictions were explained and discussed and printed material regarding diet was reviewed. Although Mr. J. was not overly responsive during these sessions, his wife demonstrated much interest and retention of information. Mrs. J. had been bringing in food from home for Mr. J. in an attempt to increase his intake of food, but after dietary restrictions were explained to her this activity ceased. He seemed to tolerate the hemodialysis treatments fairly well with only occasional complaints of headache and episodes of hypotension midway in each of the treatments. Following treatments, he experienced much gastric distress, which made food intake difficult, but he was able to retain the orally administered medications.

————————————— NURSING DIAGNOSIS —————————————

Fluid overload secondary to inadequate renal function.

Assessment

Assessment data significant to the statement of this diagnosis included:

1. A history of tight rings, shoes, and watch and reports of a slight productive cough in the morning.

2. The presence of pitting edema, ten-pound weight gain, jugular venous distention, positive hepatojugular reflex, elevated arterial pressure, and fine rales at base of lungs.

3. A serum sodium of 142 mEq/L and fine infiltrate of lung bases as seen on chest x-ray.

Plan

Intervention

Plan	Intervention	Rationale	Outcome Criteria
To achieve fluid balance.	Limit 24-hour fluid intake so that it does not exceed previous day's actual and estimated losses.	Overhydration can be prevented by balancing fluid replacement and fluid losses.	Absent jugular venous distention. Negative hepato-jugular reflex. Lungs clear. No weight gain.
	Instruct Mr. and Mrs. J. about the nature and purpose of sodium dietary restriction.	In the patient with chronic renal failure, limiting the dietary intake of sodium reduces the risk of fluid retention and thus prevents edema formation.	Serum sodium remains within normal limits. Able to list foods high in sodium. Maintains low-sodium diet.
	Administer chloro-thiazide 500 mg daily as ordered.	A specific action of the thiazide diuretic is to increase renal excretion of sodium. This action supports the reduction of edema by eliminating body sodium, which will cause passive water excretion.	Decreased pitting edema.
	Conduct hemo-dialysis treatments to remove excess fluid.	Removal of excess fluid through hemodialysis reduces circulating fluid volume and decreases the likelihood of cardiovascular complications.	Difference in pre- and post-dialysis weight reflects weight loss.

Evaluation

The interventions directed at Mr. J.'s nursing diagnosis of fluid overload were beginning to prove successful as evidenced by his overall weight reduction of seven pounds and decrease in pitting edema. However, he remained quite passive in his care and refused to take an active part in the interventions. He listened to the information that was given him regarding his diet, yet never commented or asked questions regarding his care. Although Mrs. J. was a more active listener when explanations were given, she refrained from becoming involved in any of his care. At times, she seemed angry about her husband's physical condition and confused over the complexity of her husband's care. This was evidenced by comments such as, "All the business of weighing him and checking his legs for swelling isn't really necessary, is it? I don't think I could do that at home."

NURSING DIAGNOSIS

Risk for injury to the integument associated with impaired renal function.

Assessment

Specific assessment findings upon which this diagnosis was based included:

1. History of generalized itching and reports of burning sensation along lower back, elbows, and heels following hemodialysis procedure.

2. Presence of dry, scaly skin and dependent edema, especially in legs.

Plan

Intervention

Plan	Intervention	Rationale	Outcome Criteria
To maintain integrity of skin by relieving dry skin and pruritus and stimulating circulation.	Use soap substitute for bathing.	Soaps cause increased drying of skin.	Improved appearance of skin relative to dryness and scaling.
	Apply petroleum jelly to body after bath and at bedtime.	Ointments help restore skin lubrication and impede water loss from the skin.	Skin less dry and cracked. No areas of breakdown.
	Massage bony prominences.	Prophylactic skin care measures are aimed at improving local circulation in order to maintain normal cellular homeostasis.	No evidence of circulatory impairment.
	Apply cornstarch to itching sites.	The effectiveness of this measure is found in its soothing properties to pruritic skin.	Reduction in the number and frequency of complaints of itchiness.
	Use soft brush at site of itching.	Itching is a strong sensation rarely satisfied until tissue	Fewer episodes of itching. Skin intact, without

Plan (Cont'd)	Intervention (Cont'd)	Rationale (Cont'd)	Outcome Criteria (Cont'd)
		injury or pain caused by excessive scratching occurs. Provision of a soft brush for skin stroking may be a comfort measure to the patient (Luckmann and Sorensen, 1980).	evidence of injury.
	Distract patient from focusing on the itching sensation, for example, use of TV, books, visitors.	Distraction may result in decreased attention to the itching sensation and complete cessation of the desire to scratch.	Fewer occurrences of excessive scratching.

Evaluation

The staff noted improvement in the condition of Mr. J.'s skin. Its appearance changed from dry and scaly to smooth and supple. Also, there was less flaking of skin onto the bed linen. His general complaints of itchiness decreased, and he was able to rest more soundly during the night as incidents of nocturnal itching subsided. Preventive skin care activities were effective in retarding any skin breakdown. Mr. J. remained a passive observer to most of the care that was initiated. He neither hampered the nurse in implementing medical and nursing interventions nor took an active part in starting or assisting in the delivery of care. He was appreciative of the staff's inventiveness in offering a soft brush for relief of itching. Mrs. J. was quite helpful in gathering reading material for her husband.

_____ NURSING DIAGNOSIS _____

Impaired peripheral circulation associated with diabetes mellitus.

Assessment

Assessment data upon which this diagnosis was made included the following:

1. History of intermittent claudication on walking two city blocks; pain more pronounced in left leg. Complains of having "cold feet."

2. Decreased pulses in lower extremities, more pronounced in left leg from popliteal area downward. Both legs cool to touch with slow return of

color to nail beds. Color of legs pale with a few patches of brownish discoloration. Trophic changes bilaterally. Bilateral 3+ pitting edema in lower extremities and diminished vibratory sensation.

3. Electromyography positive for peripheral nerve degeneration.

Plan

Intervention

Plan	Intervention	Rationale	Outcome Criteria
To increase peripheral blood flow.	Instruct in performing Buerger-Allen exercises.	These exercises increase collateral circulation, a necessity in patients with vascular insufficiency.	Able to carry out Buerger-Allen exercises properly.
	Encourage the wearing of socks when client complains of chilling or when chance of chilling is increased.	Insulating the feet against cold will promote vasodilatation and lessen the occurrence of reduced blood flow to the chilled part.	Fewer complaints of cold feet. Nail beds blanch with return of color in less than five seconds.

Evaluation

Although no vast improvements were noted regarding the status of Mr. J.'s peripheral circulation, no areas of tissue damage were observed either. Reports from repeat electromyography showed no change in status from the initial admission finding. He did, however, have fewer complaints of "cold feet" while wearing socks. Mr. J. carried out the Buerger-Allen exercises twice daily without any reminders from the nursing personnel. Mrs. J. remarked that he "had always taken care of himself at home" and had recently been directed by his physician to do Buerger-Allen exercises. The nursing staff felt that Mr. J.'s involvement in this aspect of his care stemmed from his previous understanding of the need for lower extremity care and the sense of environmental control obtained by making decisions about these interventions.

_____ **NURSING DIAGNOSIS** _____

Risk for infection secondary to damaged vascular system.

Assessment

Assessment data significant to the statement of this diagnosis:

1. Admits to productive cough in morning. Denies previous foot infections.

2. No cardinal signs of inflammation present; temperature 98°F orally. Hemodialysis puncture sites dry and clean. Bi-basilar rales. Lower extremities pale, cool, with decreased peripheral pulses, diminished sensation, and dependent edema.

3. Chest film shows bilateral basilar infiltrate. WBC = 8,000 cells/cu mm.

Plan

Intervention

Plan	Intervention	Rationale	Outcome Criteria
Prevent infection so as to minimize cellular disruption:			
Prevent pulmonary infection.	Turn patient and have him deep breathe every two hours.	These exercises help to maintain airway patency by mobilizing secretions, thus preventing pulmonary stasis.	Lungs clear. Chest film normal.
	Reduce number of visitors, especially ones with upper respiratory infections.	Potential for pulmonary infection decreases with limited exposure to possible contaminants.	No signs of upper respiratory infection.
Prevent A.V. fistula site infection.	Aseptic care of A.V. fistula site.	It is necessary to maintain clean A.V. fistula puncture sites, since these are access areas for entry of bacteria, which could lead to local or systemic infection.	Puncture site remains clean and dry without evidence of inflammation.
Prevent foot infection.	Wash feet daily. Apply petroleum jelly to dry areas.	Cleansing of the skin to remove pathogens and con-	No signs of tissue damage or local inflammation

Plan (Cont'd)	Intervention (Cont'd)	Rationale (Cont'd)	Outcome Criteria (Cont'd)
	Trim nails only after bathing — cut straight across and not shorter than end of toe.	taminants and lubrication and proper nail care will help to maintain tissue integrity and prevent an entry site for bacterial infection.	noted on feet. Skin less dry and cracked.

Evaluation

Mr. J. remained free from all infection at the A-V fistula site and on his feet. He was remarkably active in maintaining foot care and initiated preventive measures independently. Regarding outside visitors, Mrs. J. was asked to try to limit them, which she did by requesting that people phone or send cards instead. At first Mr. J. was not pleased with the reduced number of visitors, but as the calls and letters began to come in, he seemed to accept the restriction.

_____ **NURSING DIAGNOSIS** _____

Insufficient dietary intake associated with altered renal function.

Assessment

Assessment data significant to the formulation of this nursing diagnosis included:

1. Complaints of a loss of appetite, nausea, vomiting, sores in the mouth, and inability to eat much at meals. Mr. J. had also experienced a metallic taste and a constant feeling of unquenchable thirst.

2. Presence of gingival lesions.

3. Laboratory data revealed:
    a. Serum proteins = 4 gm per 100 ml   (normal 6.0 to 7.8 mg per 100 ml)
    b. Albumin = 2.5 gm per 100 ml   (normal 3.2 to 4.5 mg per 100 ml)
    c. Hct = 30 per cent   (normal 45 to 54 per cent)
    d. Hgb = 9 gm per 100 ml   (normal 13.5 to 18.0 gm per 100 ml)
    e. BUN = 110 mg per 100 ml   (normal 10 to 20 mg per 100 ml)

Plan

Intervention

Plan	Intervention	Rationale	Outcome Criteria
Reduce oral discomforts.	Oral hygiene at least four times a day with soft brush or swab. Rinse mouth with .25 per cent acetic acid solution.	Frequent oral hygiene with a soft brush or swabs will reduce unpleasant oral discomforts while preventing additional trauma from infection or bleeding of the gums. A weak acetic acid mouthwash solution acts to neutralize the ammonium and should result in improvement in the patient's taste sensation and relieve the urine-like breath odor (Brundage, 1976; Luckmann and Sorensen, 1980).	Fewer complaints of painful oral lesions and metallic tastes. Improved appearance in oral mucous membranes.
Increase dietary intake to maintain adequate cellular metabolism.	Serve small frequent meals.	Small frequent meals have proved to be more palatable and acceptable to the patient, thus increasing the desired nutritional intake (Brundage, 1976).	Increase in food intake. Decreased incidents of nausea and vomiting.
	Divide allowed fluid intake over a 24-hour period; offer high carbohydrate drinks.	Fluid restrictions become more acceptable to the patient when the volume of liquid available is divided over a 24-hour period, thus permitting fluid intake in response to thirst throughout an entire day. Fluid intake in the form of carbohydrate helps to reduce the rate of	Reduced complaints of thirst throughout the day. Protein levels will not decrease. BUN levels decreased.

Plan (Cont'd)	Intervention (Cont'd)	Rationale (Cont'd)	Outcome Criteria (Cont'd)
		protein catabolism and subsequent production of nitrogenous wastes (Williams, 1973; Burrell and Burrell, 1977; Brundage, 1976).	
	Elicit patient involvement in selecting dietary entrees.	By eliciting patient involvement in meal selection, the individual may feel more control regarding available food options and nutritional intake may improve.	Participates in menu selection.
	Maintain a quiet, neat environment at meal time.	In our society, eating is viewed as a social activity, with the enjoyment of food intake closely bound to the environment in which the meal is served. Meals served in a quiet, uninterrupted atmosphere are conducive to increased dietary intake and better digestion by allowing for relaxation and normal gastric motility and secretion (Luckmann and Sorensen, 1980).	Increased intake of solids from tray. Patient is able to retain food after eating without episodes of nausea or vomiting. Appearance of room at meals is improved.

Evaluation

Before the hemodialysis treatments were started, it was apparent to the staff that some of the interventions were effective in reducing the oral and gastric discomforts Mr. J. experienced. At first hesitant to cooperate in a program of frequent oral hygiene and acetic acid mouth washing, Mr. J.'s degree of participation and initiation of oral hygiene measures increased as the interventions proved effective. Dietary intake had been quite unpleasant for Mr. J., but with the introduction of small, frequent meals served in a quiet, orderly environment, he was able to eat more with less discomfort. The introduction of hemodialysis treatments made evaluation of the overall effectiveness of the interventions difficult because during the evenings following a treatment Mr. J. had severe nausea and dry heaves. He was visibly upset with the increase in discomfort he felt post dialysis. Mrs. J. was helpful to her husband during the periods of nausea and vomiting by staying with him, giving him cold compresses, talking quietly to him, and in general being supportive by her presence.

NURSING DIAGNOSIS

Anxiety related to severe and chronic alterations in health status.

Assessment

Assessment data that formed the basis for this nursing diagnosis included:

1. Admission by patient of increasing fatigue and decreased ability to concentrate.
2. Reluctance of patient to assume control in health care treatment activities.
3. Refusal of patient to consider and decide on future alternatives for health maintenance.
4. Expressions of anger by patient and spouse about health status and its treatment.
5. Knowledge that there are many sources of anxiety in chronic illness, as illustrated in Figure 13–1.

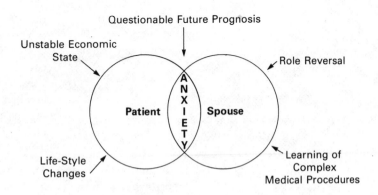

Figure 13-1 Sources of anxiety in chronic illness.

Plan

Intervention

Plan	Intervention	Rationale	Outcome Criteria
To reduce Mr. & Mrs. J.'s level of anxiety.	Provide opportunities for joint and individual conferences to encourage: a. the verbalization of feelings about Mr. J.'s illness and hospitalization;	Talking about one's feelings with others helps to temper the intensity of the emotion, which promotes insight into those feelings.	Able to verbalize their feelings to the nurse and to each other.
	b. the identification of anxiety-producing stimuli;	Before anxiety can be reduced, its sources must be identified.	Able to identify their sources of anxiety.
	c. the identification of past mechanisms used in stressful situations.	Discussion of past methods of handling stress helps to identify those which were positive and productive. Knowledge that stress has been handled productively in the past encourages a feeling of confidence in one's own inner strength (Brundage, 1976; Santopietro, 1975).	Able to identify their coping mechanisms.
	Create opportunities for Mr. J. to make decisions about aspects of his health care regime.	Making decisions about any aspect of hospitalized care promotes an individual's sense of control over the environment. Success in minor decision-making encourages one to risk a more major decision.	Decision-making activities regarding health care in the hospital increase.
	Encourage Mrs. J.'s participation in husband's care.	The spouse's involvement in patient care may lessen anxiety by increasing her sense of productivity, power, and self-confidence.	Increased self-confident involvement in patient's care.

Plan (Cont'd)	Intervention (Cont'd)	Rationale (Cont'd)	Outcome Criteria (Cont'd)
	Teach Mr. & Mrs. J. about dialysis treatment program through short information sessions, demonstrations, and written materials.	Reducing the unknown through education is an effective means to reduce anxiety. Brief teaching sessions and the provision of written materials facilitate learning when the learners are anxious (Breu and Dracup, 1978; Gardner and Stewart, 1978).	Able to paraphrase information provided and ask questions relevant to treatment program. Fewer incidents of repetitious questioning.

Evaluation

Non-communicative and non-participatory at first, Mr. and Mrs. J. gradually responded to some of the anxiety-decreasing interventions attempted by the nursing staff. Mr. J. began to discuss his feelings and reactions to this illness, how "infantile" his behavior had been when he was told he had diabetes, and how it was just easier to "let other people take care of me at first." Mr. J. could see similarities in his reaction then and his behavior now. He was able to identify some regressive behavior evidenced by his "refusal to make any decisions." Following this self-discovery of his behavior pattern, Mr. J. seemed to become more relaxed and began to talk about things that were presently worrying him — "my future health," "how will I pay the bills now that my wife lost her job and I'm only working part-time," and "what kind of life am I going to have with this dialysis." Mrs. J. began to identify her own sources of anxiety and acknowledge them to herself and her husband. Both partners became increasingly involved in Mr. J.'s care and decisions about that care. Their participation in learning about dialysis increased.

SUMMARY

Nursing of the patient with a chronic illness requires a broad theory base and understanding of the integral response mechanisms the body has to stressors. Science has shown that through the ages, man has learned to adapt to changes in environment, internal and external, in order to survive. This powerful ability is overwhelmed at times by the extent and speed with which stressors attack a system. In client situations such as Mr. J.'s, supportive health care measures are needed to enhance a person's ability to adapt. The nurse has the responsibility to assess, diagnose, plan, intervene, and evaluate situations in which the individual cannot maintain adequate compensatory responses to effect adaptation.

The nurse of today who chooses to work in a hospital setting with chronically ill patients requiring complex therapy will discover a new facet of nursing. Her skillful use of the nursing process will prepare her to intelligently assess the status of the patient and draw appropriate nursing diagnoses from the data gathered. It will facilitate her plan and initiation of interventions and allow her to cooperate in the implementation of a complex therapeutic program. Evaluation of outcomes will provide a dynamic nature to her care and afford her the opportunity to be responsbile for her professional decisions and activities. Effective use of the nursing process, then, demands that the nurse continually update her initial knowledge base to cope with the future nursing and medical innovations, the discoveries in treatment modalities, and the consequent needs that will arise in the chronically ill hospitalized adult.

References

Breu, C., and Dracup, K.: Helping the spouses of critically ill patients. *Am. J. Nurs.*, *78:*50, 1978.

Brundage, D.J.: *Nursing Management of Renal Problems*. St. Louis, The C.V. Mosby Company, 1976.

Burrell, Z.L., Jr., and Burrell, L.O.: *Critical Care*. St. Louis, The C.V. Mosby Company, 1977.

Gardner, D., and Stewart, N.: Staff involvement with families of patients in critical-care units. *Heart and Lung*, *7:*105, 1978.

Hudak, C.M., Lohr, T., and Gallo, B.: *Critical Care Nursing*. New York, J.B. Lippincott Company, 1977.

Luckmann, J. and Sorensen, K.C.: *Medical-Surgical Nursing: A Psychophysiologic Approach*. Philadelphia, W.B. Saunders Company, 1980.

Santopietro, M.S.: Meeting the emotional needs of hemodialysis patients and their spouses. *Am. J. Nurs.*, *75:*629, 1975.

Williams, S.R.: *Nutrition and Diet Therapy*. St. Louis, The C.V. Mosby Company, 1973.

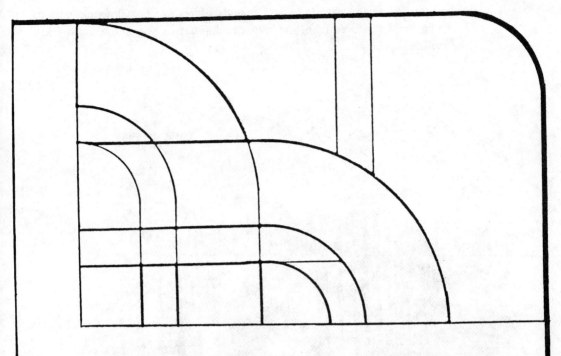

14 NURSING DIAGNOSIS AND HOME CARE OF THE AGED CLIENT

Patricia L. Demuth, R.N., Ph.D.
Dorothy E. Sassenrath, R.N., M.S.

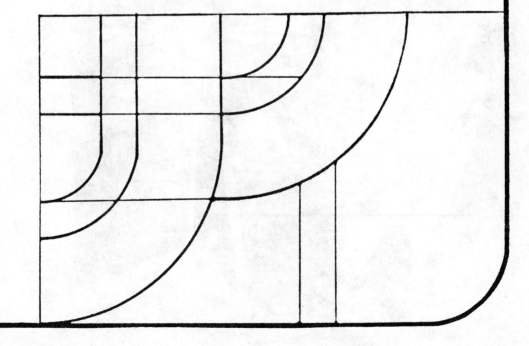

Nobody grows old by merely living a number of years. People grow old only by deserting their ideals. Years may wrinkle the skin but to give up interest wrinkles the soul.

General Douglas MacArthur

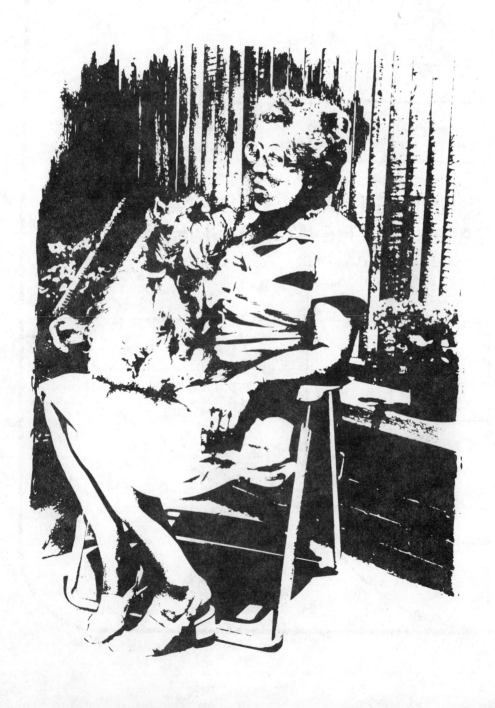

Since 1950 there has been an increase in the geriatric population, and this number will continue to increase into the year 2000. Butler (1975) emphasized the importance of the following: "Ninety-five per cent of the older poplulation live in the community with only five per cent in institutions. Eighty-one per cent are physically capable of getting around on their own with no assistance." It is this population of the aged that is the focus of this chapter. The older individual with minimal health problems who resides in the home and participates as a member of the community requires assistance at times to promote successful adaptation to the aging process. The nurse, as a member of the health team, contributes to this adaptation through the scientific approach to each step of the nursing process.

The importance of recognizing the normal physiological changes of aging as well as the psychological, cultural, social, and developmental dimensions of adaptation concomitant with these changes is of paramount importance to all nurses and all members of the health care team. The aging process manifests itself in a variety of ways as a gradual slowing and deterioration of the adaptational abilities and resources of the individual. In formulating a nursing diagnosis for an aging client, it is imperative that the nurse recognize normal aging and the changes associated with it in order to make a distinction between what is normal health and what is a deterioration of the health status (Dye and Sassenrath, 1979).

Normal aging changes are manifested as losses. Physiological losses occur in virtually every system, organ, and cell in the body in varying degrees. Examples of these losses are the loss of hearing acuity, particularly at high frequency ranges and the loss of elasticity in muscle fibers. Some of the muscles affected include those that affect the lens of the eye in visual accommodation and those of the gastrointestinal tract, which may undergo changes resulting in disturbances of digestion and elimination functions.

In the psychosocial dimension, the loss of roles that may occur with aging or disability is a frequent cause of depression in the elderly client. The roles of parent, grandparent, neighbor, housekeeper, and church member are all significant factors to be considered. Uhlenberg (1979) in his study of older women reported that ". . . the engagement of older women in constructive roles is probably the most effective means of reducing premature dependency and senility."

Another important dimension to be considered is the level of attainment of the developmental tasks of aging (Fig. 14–1). The first of these tasks is the conservation of the resources the individual has acquired throughout a lifetime of experience. Drawn from the psychosocial, economic, and educational realms, these resources include levels of health and energy as well as family, friends, and other support systems. A second developmental task is referred to as transcendence, which implies the adjustment necessary to transcend the bodily ailments and multiple physical limitations that accompany aging. The preparation and adaptation for death — both their own and the death of loved ones — is a third developmental task of the aged. The fourth task involves adjustment for and acceptance of other losses in later life whether they be social, environmental, or economic.

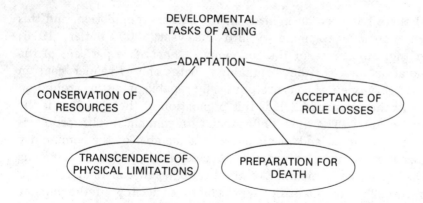

Figure 14–1   Developmental tasks of aging.

The aged have acquired a lifetime of resources that may promote or interfere with successful adaptation. A variety of support systems have been utilized including environmental, cultural, and religious. The nurse must identify the ways that the indivduals can be assisted to achieve and maintain a level of wellness relative to the limitations imposed by the altered adaptive processes.

In this chapter a model is presented to illustrate the nursing approach directed toward maintaining the aging client in the home and supporting those abilities and resources that facilitate independent living. The nursing diagnoses are derived from the nurse's assessment. Each of the selected diagnoses are followed by the plan for the nursing approach, the interventions, the outcome criteria, and the evaluation.

CLIENT SITUATION

Mrs. M. is a 78 year old widow. She is currently receiving health care through the outpatient clinic of the community hospital, which is located six miles from her home. For the past five years she has had a medical diagnosis of osteoarthritis of both hands and knees. Her history also indicated periodic episodes of early morning dizziness. The laboratory studies have remained essentially within normal limits. Her medications include acetylsalicylic acid gr $\bar{X}$ TID, indomethacin 25 mg TID, and magnesium aluminum hydroxide 30 ml with lunch and supper when necessary for gastric distress. At her last visit to the clinic, Mrs. M. related that she was having increased difficulty in mobility and expressed concern about keeping further appointments at the clinic. Consequently, the nurse practitioner was requested to visit Mrs. M. in her home for an evaluation of the home environment and health status.

The health assessment on the first home visit by the nurse practitioner revealed the following data: Mrs. M., of first generation German descent, resides alone in her home with her pet terrier "Sloopy." Mrs. M. has lived in the residential suburb of a midwestern city for the past thirty years since she and her late husband moved from Pennsylvania when he was transferred to his job on the railroad. Mr. M. died in 1974, and Mrs. M. has managed well since his death. The five-room bungalow that Mrs. M. has owned for the past ten years has been well maintained. Since the death of her husband, Mrs. M. has received assistance from neighbors in maintaining and caring for the repairs needed on her home.

Mrs. M. is a meticulous housekeeper as evidenced by the appearance of her home. She is conservative with her finances and receives a monthly check from her husband's railroad pension along with her social security benefits. She has no outstanding debts and manages her food and maintenance budget carefully. Mrs. M. is well known in the neighborhood, and there appears to be a strong indication of respect and protection toward her by the neighbors, who visit her regularly and offer much support. They have volunteered their services often and encouraged her to arrange for them to assist her with her grocery shopping.

Mrs. M. is the mother of three children, two sons and one daughter, all of whom are married and reside in other states. Her daughter moved to another city about one year ago, and Mrs. M. misses her three grandchildren with whom she was very close. She maintains contact with her daughter by weekly phone calls and writes weekly letters to all three of her children. The children and grandchildren visit her on most of the holidays.

"Sloopy" is the pet terrier who is Mrs. M.'s constant companion. After her husband's death, "Sloopy" was given as a gift from her grandchildren. She has cared for him since he was a six week old puppy. The dog sleeps in the basement, and in the past Mrs. M. took him for daily walks and romps in the backyard. He is a good watchdog and is very protective of his owner.

Participation in activities of her church have always occupied a great deal of Mrs. M.'s time and interest. She attended daily religious services and is a member of the women's organization affiliated with the church. Mrs. M. participated in quilting and needlework activities to raise funds for the organization. She prided herself in her baking and cooking for the church bazaars. In the past she enjoyed working outdoors in her flower garden. Mrs. M. has noticed that her decreased vision has disrupted her favorite hobbies of needlework and cards.

She related that she was having increased difficulty in mobility. She finds it difficult to get to the store and difficult to manage the basement stairs in her home. Mrs. M. stated that she knew the social worker had been in contact with her daughter to discuss alternate living plans for her. The topic was most upsetting to her, and she expressed concern that apartment living or nursing home placement would mean giving up so many things, especially her home, her neighbors, and "Sloopy," her pet. Mrs. M. expressed her concerns about the changes in her life style:

I went from the top down. I lost my husband. Everyone has left me — my children all moved away. I miss my grandchildren — I never see them. I was always so active, and now look at me. I cannot do my church work or anything. I was always so active, but now I get tired so easily. I have to rely on my neighbors to do my grocery shopping. I am afraid by myself because I might fall. Sloopy is my protector, and now I may have to move away and leave him.

Assessment

The following significant findings were noted on further assessment:

Temperature: 98.4°F.

Pulse: 68/min.

Respirations: 16/min.

Blood pressure: 100/78

Skin: Dry, pale, and cool. Reddened area approximately three centimeters in diameter noted on the lateral aspect of the right foot resulting from pressure of shoe.

Visual status: Acuity: 20/50 o.d., 20/30 o.s., 20/30 o.u. with glasses. Pupils: equal, round, with a slight decrease in reaction to light and accommodation. Slight yellowing of sclera of right eye. Decrease in peripheral vision noted upon examination by confrontation.

Nutrition: Height: 5'5"; weight: 98 pounds, reflecting a 10 pound loss in the past month. Poor fitting dentures. Client reports burning sensation in stomach periodically (three times within past two weeks). Expresses loss of appetite and loss of interest in meal preparation; eats irregularly; dislikes eating alone; prefers fruits and vegetables; intake of meat has decreased "because it costs too much."

Sleep patterns: Retires at 10:30 p.m.; awakens early in the morning with pain and stiffness in joints. Notes dizziness upon arising and states: "I'm afraid I might fall some morning, and then who would take care of Sloopy."

Musculoskeletal: Broad-based stance with stooped posture; gait indicates a listing to the right side with increased weight bearing on the right foot. Swelling was noted in both knees; client reported pain and stiffness in both knees, more severe on the left side; pain increased with flexion of knees; reports difficulty when ambulating. Client states: "I'm exhausted at night because it is so difficult for me to walk." The presence of Heberden's nodes on both hands and slight limitation of movement in the distal phalanges were noted.

All other assessment findings were essentially normal.

Based on the assessment completed by the nurse practitioner, nursing diagnoses were made and plans for nursing intervention and evaluation were developed. The following nursing diagnoses have been selected to be included in this chapter.

Nursing Diagnoses	*Assessment Data*
Alteration in mobility related to pain and stiffness in knees.	Pain and stiffness in both knees.
Altered nutritional status associated with loss of appetite.	Loss of appetite. 10 pound weight loss in the past month. Irregular eating habits. Lack of incentive to prepare meals. Decreased energy levels. Inability to shop for groceries. Concern over high cost of meat.
Alterations in visual perception affecting safety and activities of daily living.	Decrease in pupillary reaction to light and accommodation. Decrease in peripheral vision. Visual changes affecting color perception. Decrease in visual acuity.
At risk for injury related to dizziness with position change.	Reports of early morning dizzy spells.
Altered skin integrity related to pressure from shoe.	Reddened area (3 cm.) noted on lateral aspect of right foot. Compensatory gait.
Role losses resulting in threat to self-esteem.	Expressed concerns about: (1) Possible loss of home, pet, loss of frequent contact with family; (2) Change of life style; (3) Lack of energy to maintain activities of daily living and household responsibilities; (4) Decreased opportunities for socialization.

_____ **NURSING DIAGNOSIS** _____

Alteration in mobility related to pain and stiffness in knees.

Plan

Intervention

Plan	Intervention	Outcome Criteria
Increase mobility by decreasing pain and stiffness of knees.	Encourage warm tub baths in early morning to promote circulation and reduce swelling of knee joints.	Reports less pain and swelling during morning household activities.
	Teach Mrs. M. a plan for exercise to include range of motion of extremities three times a day with first exercise to follow bath.	Returns demonstration of exercises. No evidence of knee flexion contracture.
	Encourage altered schedule of activity to allow for: (a) rest period in morning and afternoon with knees positioned in extension;	Schedule adjusted to include one hour rest period in morning and afternoon.
	(b) balance of activities that require high expenditure of energy, for example, cooking and cleaning.	Reports more ease in completion of household duties.
	Adjust schedule of prescribed medication (indomethacin) to provide morning dose one hour prior to arising.	Reports less pain and stiffness on arising.
	Teach the proper use of a quadripod cane to reduce weight bearing on left side.	Demonstrates effective use of cane for ambulation.

Evaluation

Pain and stiffness of knee joints lessened as Mrs. M. adheres to plan for heat, exercise, and balanced plan of activity and rest. Verbalized compliance to plan and demonstrates exercise routines. Appears pleased with progress in mobility that facilitates independence in functions of daily living.

_____ **NURSING DIAGNOSIS** _____

Altered nutritional status associated with loss of appetite.

Plan

Intervention

Plan	Intervention	Outcome Criteria
Improve nutritional intake to meet metabolic demands.	Allow Mrs. M. to express her feelings about eating.	Verbalizes deterrents to eating properly.
	Explain the importance of adequate nutrition.	Expresses interest in improving her eating habits.
	Encourage six small meals per day including evening snack.	Verbalizes increased appetite and food intake. Weight gain of two pounds in two weeks (90 to 92 pounds).
	Provide simple menus and guidance for meal planning.	Diet records demonstrate improved food intake.
	Contact church members to explore the possibility of participation in activities that include meals.	Attends a church dinner with neighbor.
	Arrange for homemaker service to provide transportation for grocery shopping.	Homemaker assists with grocery shopping.

Evaluation

Increased interest and performance in meal preparation noted since Mrs. M. has been able to shop. Appetite improved with two pound weight gain in two weeks. Expresses ability to accomplish household tasks with less exhaustion.

_____ **NURSING DIAGNOSIS** _____

Alterations in visual perception affecting safety and activities of daily living.

Plan

Intervention

Plan	Intervention	Outcome Criteria
Develop an approach to promote adaptation to visual changes related to: decreased peripheral vision, diminished color discrimination, light accommodation, and visual acuity.	Teach Mrs. M. about the effect of visual changes related to aging. Modify environment to accommodate for decrease in peripheral vision by reorganization of essential items for activities of daily living.	Cabinets reorganized in the bathrooms and kitchen so that items used daily are clearly visible.
	Encourage use of bright colors to accommodate for loss of color discrimination.	Feedback from client indicates a knowledge of the importance and use of bright colors as well as the importance of improved lighting for safety.
	Adapt phone dial with large print.	Dial obtained. Calls neighbors daily.
	Increase lighting in halls and place night lights in bedroom, stairwells, and hallway.	Uses increased lighting at night and when sewing.
	Arrange for eye examination.	Appointment scheduled for two weeks.

Evaluation

Adaptations in Mrs. M.'s home environment through the use of increased lighting and removal of rugs and furniture that were safety hazards have improved her ability to perform activities of daily living. An eye appointment has been scheduled for a review of the status of her vision and possible change in lenses.

_____ NURSING DIAGNOSIS _____

At risk for injury related to dizziness with position change.

Plan

Intervention

Plan	Intervention	Outcome Criteria
Alter activities that may contribute to "dizziness."	Teach Mrs. M. the importance of (1) Changing position gradually from horizontal to vertical position when arising from the bed. (2) Avoiding bending over, rotating the head quickly, hyperextending the head, and standing immediately after eating.	Reports no episodes of dizziness when position changes are carried out as instructed.

Evaluation

Mrs. M. verbalizes her understanding of the relationship of position change to dizziness. Protocol for pacing of activities with position change has eliminated the incidents of early morning dizziness.

_____ NURSING DIAGNOSIS _____

Altered skin integrity related to pressure from shoe.

Plan

Intervention

Plan	Intervention	Outcome Criteria
Promote healing and prevent further tissue damage to foot by eliminating the sources contributing to pressure and tissue damage.	Encourage warm water soaks BID followed by elevation of extremity.	Reduction of reddened area from 3 cm to 2 cm.
Correction of gait pattern to reduce weight-bearing pressure on right side.	Provide instruction related to proper gait and weight-bearing techniques.	Demonstrates equal distribution of weight bearing when walking.
	Provide information and referral for the selection of proper fitting shoes.	Plans are made for transportation to purchase proper shoes.

Evaluation

Improvement in pressure area of right foot has occurred as evidenced by reduction in size of the reddened area and observation of tissue healing. Relief of pain in knees has eliminated compensatory gait and relieved pressure. Ambulation has improved with equal distribution of weight. Fitting with proper shoes should prevent further skin damage.

--- **NURSING DIAGNOSIS** ---

Role losses resulting in threat to self-esteem.

Plan

Intervention

Plan	Intervention	Outcome Criteria
Diminish impact of perceived losses.	Provide time and opportunities for client to verbalize and identify perceived losses. Reassure Mrs. M. relative to fears about loss of home, pet, and family.	Discusses concerns openly.
	Explore with Mrs. M. ways to alter living arrangements to minimize losses and promote independence.	Accepts suggestions for alteration of life style.
	Arrange for meeting with client, daughter, and social worker to explore necessary alterations in life style.	Meeting arranged.
	Explore homemaker services to provide for assistance in grocery shopping, cleaning, and transportation.	Weekly visits arranged.
	Consult with church members and clergy regarding available volunteer services.	Arrangements made for frequent visits and transportation to church and church-related activities.
	Consult with occupational therapist at the local Chapter of the Arthritis Foundation for available services.	Plans in progress to work with client through assistance of occupational therapist for evaluation of home environment to promote adaptation.

Plan (Cont'd)	Intervention (Cont'd)	Outcome Criteria (Cont'd)
Reactivate social contacts.	Arrange participation in local programs with Elementary School Children Visitors.	Verbalization of satisfaction with school childrens' visits.
	Explore available sources of organized senior citizen activities in the community.	Selects two activities weekly of senior citizen program.
	Develop a plan with client for assistance in caring for "Sloopy."	Arrangements have been completed for neighbor's son to walk the dog each day.

Evaluation

Discussion between Mrs. M., her family, and the nurse resulted in resolution of threats to client's self-esteem. Plans for a change in life style that would decrease the loss of independent roles for the client were outlined and accepted by the client. Social contacts have been reestablished, and "Sloopy" remains a member of the household. Assistance with shopping and household activities have enabled client to maintain independence within the home for the present.

SUMMARY

In this chapter, the importance of nursing diagnosis for the elderly client is described as an essential component of the nursing process. Subsequent to analysis and classification of assessment data, the case study describes the use of nursing diagnosis to establish a plan of care that would support the strengths of the elderly client in her goal for independent living within the home environment. Nursing interventions and outcome criteria were specified that would achieve the nursing plan for Mrs. M. While the future plans for Mrs. M. may take a different course, it is hoped that, for the present, she will regain a degree of independence. Such freedom will permit her to continue to live independently and at peace within her home and with her supportive pet terrier, who may well be the major contributing factor to a successful plan of care.

References:

Butler, R.N.: *Why Survive? Being Old in America.* New York, Harper and Row Publishers, Inc., 1975.

Dye, C., and Sassenrath, D.: Identification of normal aging and disease related processes by health care professionals. *Journal of the American Geriatric Society, 27:*472, 1979.

Uhlenberg, P.: Older women: The growing challenge to design constructive roles. *The Gerontologist, 19:*241, 1979.

General References

Abramson, D.: *Vascular Disorders of the Extremities*, 2nd ed. Hagerstown, Maryland, Harper and Row, 1974.

Adaptation: A Theoretical Base for Nursing. St. Louis University School of Nursing, Unpublished, 1979.

Alberti, R., and Emmons, M.: *Your Perfect Right*, 3rd ed. San Luis Obispo, Impact Co., 1978.

Anderson, B.: Nursing by trial and error — The standard misconception. *Supervisor Nurse*, 7:35, 1976.

Anderson, N.: An interactive systems approach to problem solving. *Nurse Practitioner*, 3:25, 1978.

Andreoli, K., Fowkes, V., Zipes, D., and Wallace, A.: *Comprehensive Cardiac Care*, 4th ed. St. Louis, The C.V. Mosby Co., 1979.

Annon, J.: *Behavioral Treatment of Sexual Problems.* Honolulu, Enabling Systems Co., 1975.

Aspinall, M.J.: Nursing diagnosis — The weak link. *Nursing Outlook, 24:*433, 1976.

Balag, T.G.: A mother's reaction to diagnosis of congenital anomalies in her child. *Maternal-Child Nursing Journal, 1*:143, 1972.

Barnoon, S., and Wolfe, H.. *Measuring the Effectiveness of Medical Decisions.* Springfield, Charles C Thomas, 1972.

Becvar, R.: *Skills for Effective Communication: A Guide to Building Relationships.* New York, John Wiley and Sons, Inc., 1974.

Beland, I.: *Clinical nursing — Pathophysiological and Psychosocial Approaches*, 3rd ed. London, Macmillan Co., 1975.

Benson, H.: *The Relaxation Response.* New York, The Hearst Corporation, 1975.

Berg, A.: Prevention in perspective: History, concepts and issues. *Journal of Family Practice, 9:*37, 1979.

Bergman, J., and Werblin, M.: Chronic pain — A review. *Journal of Family Practice*, 7:685, 1978.

Bevis, E.O.: *Curriculum Building in Nursing*, 2nd ed. St. Louis, The C.V. Mosby Co., 1978.

Bininger, C.J., and Kisel, Sr., M.: Assessment of perceived role losses in the gerian. *Journal of Gerontological Nursing, 4:*24, 1978.

Bircher, A.U.: On the development and classification of diagnoses. *Nursing Forum, 14:*10, 1975.

Bishop, B.: A guide to assessing parenting capabilities. *American Journal of Nursing, 76:*1784, 1976.

Blair, C., and Salerno, E.: *The Expanding Family: Childbearing.* Boston, Little, Brown & Company, 1976.

Bonica, J.: *Principles and Practice of Obstetric Analgesia and Anesthesia:* Philadelphia, F.A. Davis, 1972.

Brewer, T.: Human maternal fetal nutrition. *American Journal of Obstetrics and Gynecology, 40:*868, 1972.

Brown, M.: The epidemiologic approach to the study of clinical nursing diagnoses. *Nursing Forum, 13:*346, 1974.

Burch, G., and Giles, T.: Alcoholic cardiomyopathy. *American Journal of Medicine, 50:*141, 1971.

Burnside, I.M. (ed.): *Psychosocial Care of the Aged.* New York, McGraw-Hill Book Company, 1980.

Burnside, I.M., Ebersole, P., and Monea, H.E. (eds.): *Psychosocial Caring Throughout the Life Span.* New York, McGraw-Hill Book Company, 1979.

Buseck, S.A.: Visual status of the elderly. *Journal of Gerontological Nursing, 2:*34, 1976.

Busse, E.W.: How mind, body and environment influence nutrition in the elderly. *Postgraduate Medicine, 63:*118, 1978.

Butler, R., and Lewis, M.: *Aging and Mental Health: Positive Psychosocial Approaches*, 2nd ed. St. Louis, The C.V. Mosby Company, 1977.

Carnevali, D.L., and Patrick, M. (eds.): *Nursing Management for the Elderly*. Philadelphia, J.B. Lippincott Company, 1979.

Carrieri, V.K., and Sitzman, J.: Components of the nursing process. *Nursing Clinics of North America, 6:*115, 1971.

Chambers, W.: Nursing diagnosis. *American Journal of Nursing, 62:*102, 1962.

Closurdo, J.: Behavior modification and the nursing process. *Perspectives in Psychiatric Care, 13:*25, 1975.

Coates, J: Obstetrics in the very young adolescent. *American Journal of Obstetrics, 108*: 68, 1970.

Cohen, B., Ball, W., Brasheain, S., et al.: Risk factors in chronic obstructive pulmonary disease. *American Journal of Epidemiology, 105:*223, 1977.

Comfort, A.: *A Good Age.* New York, Crown Publishers, Inc., 1976.

Conte, A., Brandzel, M., and Whitehead, S.: Group work with hypertensive patients. *American Journal of Nursing, 74:*910, 1974.

Cospers, B.: The yoyo factor in chronic illness. *Nursing Forum, 13:*207, 1974.

Danforth, D. (ed.): *Textbook of Obstetrics and Gynecology*, 3rd ed. New York, Harper and Row, 1977.

Diagnostic titles. The Clearinghouse — National Group for Classification of Nursing Diagnosis, St. Louis University School of Nursing, St. Louis, 1977.

Doona, M.E.: The judgment process in nursing. *Image, 13:*27, 1976.

Eddy, M.E.: Teaching patients with peripheral vascular disease. *Nursing Clinics of North America, 12:*151, 1977.

Eddy, T.P.: Nutritional needs of the old. *Nursing Times, 70:*1499, 1974.

Ehmann, V.: Empathy: Its origin, characteristics and process. *Perspectives of Psychiatric Care, 9:*72, 1971.

Erikson, E.H.: *Childhood and Society*, 2nd ed. New York, Norton & Company, 1963.

Erikson, F.: Nursing care based on nursing assessment. *In* E.H. Anderson, B.S. Bergerson, M. Duffey, and M.H. Rose (eds.): *Current Concepts in Clinical Nursing*, Vol. 2. St. Louis, The C.V. Mosby Company, 1969.

Evans, F.: *Psychosocial Nursing: Theory and Practice in Hospital and Community Health.* New York, Macmillan Company, 1971.

Faterson, H., and Witkin, H.: Longitudinal study of development of the body concept. *Developmental Psychology, 2:*429, 1970.

Feinstein, A.R.: *Clinical Judgment.* Baltimore, Williams & Wilkins, 1967.

Fink, J.: The asthmatic. *American Family Physician, 18:*124, 1978.

Finnerty, F., Mattie, E., and Finnerty III, F.: Hypertension in the inner city — Analysis of clinic dropouts. *Circulation, 47:*73, 1973.

Fisher, S.: A further appraisal of the body boundary concept. *Journal of Consulting Psychology, 28:*62, 1963.

Fisher, S., and Cleveland, S.: *Body Image and Personality*, 2nd ed. New York, Dover Publications, 1968.

Francis, G.: Loneliness: Measuring the abstract. *Int. Journal of Nursing Studies, 13:*153, 1976.

Gaitz, C.M., and Baer, P.E.: Diagnostic assessment of the elderly: A multifunctional model. Part 1. *The Gerontologist, 10:*47, 1970.

Gardner, D., and Stewart, N.: Staff involvement with families of patients in critical-care units. *Heart and Lung, 1:*105, 1978.

Gebbie, K.M. (ed.): *Classification of Nursing Diagnoses — Summary of the Second National Conference.* St. Louis, The Clearinghouse — National Group for Classification of Nursing Diagnoses, 1976.

Gebbie, K.M., and Lavin, M.A.: Classifying nursing diagnoses. *American Journal of Nursing, 74:*250, 1974.

Gebbie, K.M., and Lavin, M.A. (eds.): *Classification of Nursing Diagnoses — Proceedings of the First National Conference.* St. Louis, The C.V. Mosby Co., 1975.

Geertsma, R., and Mackie, J. (eds.): *Studies in Self Cognition: Techniques of Videotape Self-Observation in the Behavioral Sciences.* Baltimore, Williams & Wilkins Co., 1969.

Gergen, K.: Multiple identity. *Psychology Today, 5:*31, 1972.

Gillespie, B., and Dandy, R.: *Counselor Training: Short Term Client Systems.* Maryland, National Institute for Drug Abuse, 1977.

Given, C., Given, B., and Simon, L.: The association of knowledge and perception of medications with compliance and health states among hypertension patients. *Research in Mental Health, 1:*76, 1978.

Gordon, M.: *Information Processing Strategies in Nursing Diagnosis.* Unpublished paper, 1972.

Gordon, M.: Nursing diagnosis and the diagnostic process. *American Journal of Nursing, 76:*1298, 1976.

Gordon, M.: The concept of nursing diagnosis. *Nursing Clinics of North America, 14:*487, 1979.

Gruis, M.: Beyond maternity: Postpartum concerns of mothers. *American Journal of Maternal Child Nursing, 2:*182, 1977.

Gunn, G., Mishell, D., and Morton, D.: Premature rupture of the fetal membranes. *American Journal of Obstetrics and Gynecology, 106:*469, 1970.

Hale, S., and Richardson, J.: Terminating the nurse-patient relationship. *American Journal of Nursing, 63:*116, 1963.

Hardgrove, C.: Living-in accommodations and practices for parents in hospital pediatric units: An update. *Journal of the Association for the Care of Children in Hospitals, 4:*24, 1975.

Hartmann, E.: *The Functions of Sleep.* New Haven and London, Yale University Press, 1973.

Hefferin, E.A., and Hunter, R.E.: Nursing assessment and care plan statements. *Nursing Research, 24:*360, 1975.

Helgeson, D., and Newburger, Sr., C.: Maintaining and supporting health and wellness during pregnancy. *Health Values, 1:*108, 1977.

Henderson, B.: Nursing diagnosis: Theory and practice. *Advances in Nursing Science, 1:*75, 1978.

Herbert, V., et al.: Folic acid deficiency in the United States: Folate assays in a prenatal clinic. *American Journal of Obstetrics and Gynecology, 123*(2):175, 1975.

Hess, P., and Day, C.: *Understanding the Aging Patient.* Bowie, Maryland, The Robert J. Brady Company, 1977.

Hickey, T.: Psychologic rehabilitation for the "normal" elderly. *Mental Hygiene, 53:*364, 1969.

Hightower, N., and Janowitz, H.: Biliary secretion. *In* J. Broback (ed.): *Best and Taylor's Physiological Basis of Medical Practice,* 10th ed. Baltimore, Williams & Wilkins, 1979.

Hollender, J.: Sex differences in sources of social self esteem. *Journal of Consulting and Clinical Psychology, 38:*343, 1972.

Houser, D.: What to do first when a patient complains of chest pain. *Nursing, 6:*4, 1976.

Hudak, C.M., Gallo, B.M., and Lohr, T.: *Critical Care Nursing.* Philadelphia, J.B. Lippincott Company, 1973.

Jacquez, J. (ed.): *The Diagnostic Process.* Ann Arbor, Malloy Lithographing, Inc., 1964.

Joe, V.: Review of the internal-external control construct as a personality variable. *Psychological Reports, 28:*619, 1971.

Jones, J.: Deprivation and existence or stimulation and life: Our choice for the elderly. *Journal of Gerontological Nursing, 2:*17, 1976.

Jourard, S.: *The Transparent Self.* New York, Van Nostrand Co., 1964.

Jourard, S., and Secord, P.: Body cathexis and the ideal female figure. *Journal of Abnormal and Social Psychology, 50:*243, 1955

Joyce, A., and Krawczyk, R.: Preventive nursing intervention with the elderly. *Journal of Gerontological Nursing, 4:*28, 1978.

Judge, R.D., and Zuidema, G.D. (eds.): *Physical Diagnosis: A Physiological Approach to the Clinical Examination,* 2nd ed. Boston, Little, Brown and Company, 1968.

Kalisch, B.: Strategies for developing nurse empathy. *Nursing Outlook, 19:*714, 1971.

Kalisch, B.: What is empathy? *American Journal of Nursing, 73:*1548, 1973.

Kannel, W.: Recent findings of the Framingham study. *Medical Times 106*(4):23, 1978.

Kaplan, L.: *Foundations of Human Behavior.* New York, Harper and Row, 1965.

Karmel, M.: *Thank you, Dr. Lamaze.* New York, J.B. Lippincott Company, 1959.

Kart, C.S., Metress, E.S., and Metress, J.F.: *Aging and Health: Biologic and Social Perspectives.* Menlo Park, California, Addison-Wesley Publishing Company, 1978.

King, L.: What is a diagnosis? *JAMA, 202:*714, 1967.

King, P.A.: Foot assessment of the elderly. *Journal of Gerontological Nursing, 4:*47, 1978.

Kitowski, V.: Cardiovascular disease — Prevention and rehabilitation. *Cardiovascular Diseases Bulletin of the Texas Heart Institute,* December, 1978, 418–423.

Komorita, N.: Nursing diagnosis. *American Journal of Nursing, 63:*83, 1963.

Koos, E.L.: Class differences in family reactions to crisis. *Marriage and Family Living, 12:*43, 1950.

Kopp, L.: Ordeal or ideal — The second stage of labor. *American Journal of Nursing, 71:*1140, 1971.

Kritek, P.: The generation and classification of nursing diagnoses: Toward a theory of nursing. *Image, 10:*33, 1978.

Lambert, V., and Lambert, C.: *The Impact of Physical Illness and Related Mental Health Concepts.* Englewood Cliffs, New Jersey, Prentice-Hall, Inc., 1979.

Larkin, P.D., and Backer, B.A.: *Problem-Oriented Nursing Assessment.* New York, McGraw-Hill Book Company, 1977.

Lawton, M.P.: The functional assessment of elderly people. *Journal of the American Geriatric Society, 19:*465, 1971.

Lawton, M., Powell, M., and Yaffe, S.: Mortality, morbidity and voluntary change of residence by older people. *Journal of The American Geriatric Society, 18:*823, 1970.

Leininger, M.: *Transcultural Nursing: Concepts, Theories and Practices.* New York, John Wiley and Sons, 1977.

Levinson, B.M.: Pets and old age. *Mental Hygiene, 53:*364, 1969.

Liggins, M. (ed.): Counseling for common sexual problems. *Patient Care, 10:*59, 1976.

Little, D.E., and Carnevali, D.: *Nursing Care Planning,* 2nd ed. Philadelphia, J.B. Lippincott Co., 1976.

Lowen, A.: *The Betrayal of the Body.* New York, Macmillan Company, 1969.

Luce, G.: *Biological Rhythms in Psychiatry and Medicine.* Washington, D.C., National Institute of Mental Health, 1970.

Lyskin, G.: *Parent-Child Nursing,* 2nd ed. St. Louis, The C.V. Mosby Company, 1978.

Maas, M., Specht, J., and Jacox, A.: Nurse autonomy: Reality not rhetoric. *American Journal of Nursing, 75:*2201, 1975.

Mahoney, E.A.: Some implications for nursing diagnoses of pain. *Nursing Clinics of North America, 12:*613, 1977.

Maloney, R.: Helping your hypertensive patients live longer. *Nursing '78, 8:*26, 1978.

Marston, M.: Compliance with medical regimens — A review of the literature. *Nursing Research, 19:*312, 1970.

Mayer, J.: Aging and nutrition. *Geriatrics, 29:*57, 1974.

McCaffery, M.: *Nursing Management of the Patient with Pain.* Philadelphia, J.B. Lippincott Company, 1972.

McDaniel, J.: *Physical Disability and Human Behavior,* 2nd ed. New York, Pergamon Press, 1976.

Mereness, D. : Your self image and your practice. *American Journal of Nursing, 66:*96, 1966.

Meyer, R., and Morris, D.: Alcoholic cardiomyopathy: A nursing approach. *Nursing Research, 26:*422, 1977.

Mitchell, C.: Identifying the hazard — The key to crisis intervention. *American Journal of Nursing, 77:*1194, 1977.

Mitchell, P.H. (ed.): *Concepts Basic to Nursing,* 2nd ed. New York, McGraw-Hill Book Company, 1977.

Mundinger, M.O., and Jauron, G.D.: Developing a nursing diagnosis. *Nursing Outlook, 23:*94, 1975.

Murray, R.: Principles of nursing intervention for the adult patient with body image changes. *Nursing Clinics of North America*, 7:697, 1972.

Murray, R.B., Zentner, J.P., et al.: *Nursing Assessment and Health Promotion Through the Life Span*, 2nd ed. Englewood Cliffs, N.J., Prentice-Hall, Inc., 1979.

O'Dell, A.J.: Hot packs for morning joint stiffness. *American Journal of Nursing*, 75:686, 1975.

O'Leary, K., and Wilson, G.: *Behavior Therapy*. Englewood Cliffs, New Jersey, Prentice-Hall, Inc., 1975.

Omwakee, K.: The relation between acceptance of self and acceptance of others shown by three personality inventories. *Journal of Consulting Psychology*, 18:443, 1954.

Parad, H. (ed.): *Crisis Intervention: Selected Readings*. New York, Family Service Association of America, 1965.

Petty, T. (ed.): *The Asthmatic in Trouble*. Greenwich, Connecticut, Upjohn Co., 1976.

Pierpoint, G.: Congestive cardiomyopathy: Pathophysiology and response to therapy. *Archives of Internal Medicine*, 138:1847, 1978.

Plummer, A.: Choosing a drug regimen for obstructive pulmonary disease. *Postgraduate Medicine*, 63:113, 1978.

Pollak, O.: *Human Behavior and the Helping Professions*. New York, Spectrum Publications, Inc., 1976.

Pratt, M.A.: Physical exercise: A special need in long term care. *Journal of Gerontological Nursing*, 4:38, 1978.

Puder, B.: What you should know about nursing diagnosis. *Medical Record News*, 46:87, 1975.

Redman, B.: *The Process of Patient Teaching in Nursing*, 3rd ed. St. Louis, The C.V. Mosby Company, 1976.

Reinhardt, A.M., and Quinn, M.: *Current Practice in Gerontological Nursing*. St. Louis, The C.V. Mosby Company, 1979.

Resler, M.M., and Viamontes, C.: *Nursing assessment — Outline for data collection*. Unpublished, St. Louis, 1978.

Riehl, J., and Roy, Sr., C.: *Conceptual Models for Nursing Practice*. New York, Appleton-Century-Crofts, 1974.

Rosenthal, G.K.: Achieving a healthier more hopeful old age. *Outlook Magazine*, St. Louis, Washington University School of Medicine, 16:1, 1979.

Rothberg, J.: Why nursing diagnosis? *American Journal of Nursing*, 67:1040, 1967.

Roy, Sr., C.: The impact of nursing diagnosis. *AORN Journal*, 21:1023, 1975.

Rubel, M.: Coming to grips with the nursing process. *Supervisor Nurse*, 7:30, 1976.

Rubin, R.: Basic maternal behavior. *Nursing Outlook*, 9:683, 1961.

Rubin, R.: Body image and self-esteem. *Nursing Outlook*, 16:20, 1968.

Rubin, R.: Maternity nursing stops too soon. *American Journal of Nursing*, 75:1680, 1975.

Sana, J., and Judge, R. (eds.): *Physical Appraisal Methods in Nursing Practice*. Boston, Little, Brown and Company, 1975.

Santopietro, M., and Charles, S.: Meeting the emotional needs of hemodialysis patients and their spouses. *American Journal of Nursing*, 75:629, 1975.

Saxton, D., and Hyland, P.: *Planning and Implementing Nursing Intervention*. St. Louis, The C.V. Mosby Company, 1975.

Saxton, S.V., and Etten, M.J.: *Physical Change and Aging. A Guide for Helping Professions*. New York, The Tiresias Press, 1978.

Schilder, P.: *Image and Appearance of the Human Body*. New York, International Universities Press, 1958.

Schrock, M.M.: *Holistic Assessment of the Healthy Aged*. New York, John Wiley and Sons, 1980.

Schwab, Sr., M.: Caring for the aged. *American Journal of Nursing*, 73:2049, 1973.

Shannon-Babitz, M.: Addressing the needs of fathers during labor and delivery. *The American Journal of Maternal-Child Nursing*, 14:378, 1979.

Sheehy, G.: *Passages*. New York, E.P. Dutton, 1976.

Shoemaker, J.: How nursing diagnosis helps focus your care. *R.N.*, 42:56, 1979.

Solnit, A.J., and Stark, M.H.: Mourning the birth of a defective child. *The Psychoanalytic Study of the Child*, *16*:523, 1967.

Sorensen, K.C., and Luckmann, J.: *Basic Nursing: A Psychophysiological Approach.* Philadelphia, W.B. Saunders Company, 1979.

Stevens, B.J.: ANA standards of nursing practice: What they tell us about the state of the art. *Journal of Nursing Administration*, *4*(5):16, 1974.

Sutton, M.: Management of conflict. *A.O.R.N.*, *23*:1093, 1976.

Thralow, J.U., and Watson, C.G.: Remotivation for geriatric patients using elementary school students. *The American Journal of Occupational Therapy*, *28:*469, 1974.

Townsend, P.: *Family Life of Old People.* London, Toutledge, 1957.

Travelbee, J.: *Intervention in Psychiatric Nursing.* Philadelphia, F.A. Davis Company, 1969.

Turpeinen, O.: Effect of cholesterol-lowering diet on mortality from coronary heart disease and other causes. *Circulation*, *59:*1, 1979.

Vander Zyl, S.: Psychosocial theories of aging: Activity, disengagement and continuity. *Journal of Gerontological Nursing*, *5:*45, 1979.

Vang, K.: *Promoting Health in the Human Environment.* Geneva, WHO, 1975.

Wiggins, J.D.: *Childbearing: Physiology, Experiences, Needs.* St. Louis, The C.V. Mosby Company, 1979.

Williams, B., and Richards, S.: Fetal monitoring during labor. *American Journal of Nursing*, *70:*2384, 1970.

Williams, L.: A concept of loneliness in the elderly. *Journal of the American Geriatric Society*, *26:*183, 1978.

Yunek, M., and Lojek, R.: Intrapartal fetal monitoring. *American Journal of Nursing*, *78:*2102, 1978.

Yura, H., and Walsh, M.B.: *The Nursing Process*, 3rd ed. New York, Appleton-Century-Crofts, 1978.

Zion, L.: Body concept as it relates to self concept. *The Research Quarterly*, *36:*490, 1964.

Zohman, L.: *Beyond Diet — Exercise Your Way to Health.* New York, CPC International Corporation, 1974.

INDEX

Page numbers in *italics* indicate illustrations. Page numbers followed by (t) indicate tables.